Reifying Women's Experiences with Invisible Illness

Lexington Studies in Health Communication

Series Editors: Leandra H. Hernández and Kari Nixon

National and international governments have recognized the importance of widespread, timely, and effective health communication, as research shows that accurate, patient-centered, and culturally competent health communication can improve patient and community health care outcomes. This interdisciplinary series examines the role of health communication in society and is receptive to manuscripts and edited volumes that use a variety of theoretical, methodological, interdisciplinary, and intersectional approaches. We invite contributions on a variety of health communication topics including but not limited to health communication in a digital age; race, gender, ethnicity, class, physical abilities, and health communication; critical approaches to health communication; feminisms and health communication; LGBTQIA health; interpersonal health communication perspectives; rhetorical approaches to health communication; organizational approaches to health communication; health campaigns, media effects, and health communication; multicultural approaches to health communication; and international health communication. This series is open to contributions from scholars representing communication, women's and gender studies, public health, health education, discursive analyses of medical rhetoric, and other disciplines whose work interrogates and explores these topics. Successful proposals will be accessible to an interdisciplinary audience, advance our understanding of contemporary approaches to health communication, and enrich our conversations about the importance of health communication in today's health landscape.

Recent Titles in the Series

Reifying Women's Experiences with Invisible Illness: Illusions, Delusions, Reality edited by Kesha Morant Williams and Frances Selena Morant

When the Procedures Don't Stop: Narrative Explorations of Pediatric Patients' Sense-making of Difficult and Traumatic Medical Experiences by Heather A. Hamilton-Stilwell

The Rhetoric of Breast Cancer: Patient-to-Patient Discourse in an Online Community by Carie S. Tucker King

Reifying Women's Experiences with Invisible Illness

Illusions, Delusions, Reality

Edited by Kesha Morant Williams
and Frances Selena Morant

LEXINGTON BOOKS
Lanham • Boulder • New York • London

Published by Lexington Books
An imprint of The Rowman & Littlefield Publishing Group, Inc.
4501 Forbes Boulevard, Suite 200, Lanham, Maryland 20706
www.rowman.com

Unit A, Whitacre Mews, 26-34 Stannary Street, London SE11 4AB

British Library Cataloguing in Publication Information Available

Library of Congress Cataloging-in-Publication Data Available
Library of Congress Control Number: 2017955515

∞™ The paper used in this publication meets the minimum requirements of American National Standard for Information Sciences Permanence of Paper for Printed Library Materials, ANSI/NISO Z39.48-1992.

Printed in the United States of America

Contents

Foreword

Communicating from/as/with the Body

Laura L. Ellingson

This outstanding collection of narratives of living with invisible illness transcends categories—interpretive health communication research on invisible illness, evocative autoethnography and narrative sense making, feminist and anti-racist analysis of embodied being, and incisive commentary on the culture and constraints of academic workplaces. The editor and authors refuse trite and simple accounts and instead contemplate the complex and shifting realities of daily life with invisible illness.

The editors and their contributors explore communication surrounding health and illness by grounding communication in the visceral bodies of those who produce and are produced by cultural discourses of health, illness, health care, and work (Ellingson, 2017). They approach invisible illness as an opportunity for tracking a set of trickster chronic conditions, ones that wax and wane and remain largely invisible, other than to those who suffer from them and their intimate companions. The issue of visibility is a problematic and value-laden one, for as many critical theorists have argued, we come to see that which we are trained to see (e.g., Haraway, 1988). By extension, we also fail to see what we have been carefully trained not to see, such as white people who are trained not to see the devastating effects of white privilege and systemic racism (Allen, 2010). Likewise, those in good health, who have not sustained significant injury or life-threatening illness, studiously ignore subtle signs of embodied suffering by members of the "community of pain," fostering a culture of concealment (Frank, 1995). Since overt displays of bodily failures are deeply stigmatizing (Goffman, 1959), people with chronic illness often go to great lengths to conceal or minimize the embodied signs of their illnesses, as these authors courageously document in painstaking detail.

Narrative sense making offers a vibrant qualitative and critical complement to more rigid approaches to health communication on scholarship that feature quantitative theory testing and systematic pattern analysis (Geist-Martin, Sharf, and Yamasaki, 2017; Harter, 2013). Autoethnography and personal narratives illuminate individual experiences, demonstrating the "*radical specificity* of living a life, not in the sense that we all live our own lives but in the sense that life is lived in the flows, multiplicities, and provisionality of each moment, event, emotion" (Sotirin, 2010, n.p., original emphasis). The authors go beyond simply documenting their personal experiences in navigating invisible illness to illuminate moments of living as bodies-in-relation with others and the exquisite pains, pleasures, and possibilities that brings.

Taken together, the chapters also offer a critique of power and agency in health care for people with chronic illnesses. Each of these women's struggles to manage medications (and side effects) and other treatments, cope with symptoms, coordinate with physicians and other health care providers, and navigate the (in)visibility of their illness with colleagues, friends, and family shows how exhausting this daily process can be. Further, these experiences reflect the gendered and racial realities of chronic illness, where women typically bear higher treatment burden and caregiver burden than do men (Sav, King, Whitty, Kendall, McMillan, Kelly... and Wheeler, 2015), the intersectionality of gender and race reflects a greater burden of chronic illnesses on communities of color (e.g., Bauer, Briss, Goodman, and Bowman, 2014).

In the midst of their ambitious project of illuminating the complexities of invisible illness, the collaborators also illustrate both opportunities and constraints of academia as a workplace, since that is where the first editor and many of the authors work (Bloch, 2016). Paradoxically, the academy is both extremely flexible and not at all flexible for faculty members. On the one hand, when scheduling courses, research, and service, faculty hours are generally flexible to accommodate preferences for teaching earlier or later in the day, in more concentrated bursts or distributed in shorter periods, and the ability to attend medical appointments, at least in comparison to a traditional office position. Moreover, much academic work can be completed at home or otherwise outside of a university office and standard work hours. On the other hand, the centuries old tenure system flexes very little to accommodate illnesses. While leaves and tenure clock extensions for child bearing and some types of illnesses have become more common, the urgent need to publish within a tightly defined period of time while also establishing one's efficacy as a teacher and committee member is challenging enough before the toll taken by chronic illness.

Finally, I would like to offer a personal perspective on this collection. As a white, female professor and a cancer survivor who lives with chronic phantom limb pain and significant side effects of pain medications, I was deeply moved by the courage of each author to make visible and public that which she has tried for so long to manage invisibly or at least inconspicuously in her daily life. Again and again, I resonated with the feelings of fear, shame, resentment, fatigue, and (occasional) satisfaction expressed by the authors—"me, too!" I said aloud, over and over again (Mairs, 1997). The power of passion and creativity to survive—and even have moments of thriving—in the academy with an invisible illness was affirmed for me, bridging my personal and professional spheres.

REFERENCES

Allen, B. J. (2010). *Difference matters: Communicating social identity*. Long Grove, IL: Waveland Press.

Bauer, U. E., Briss, P. A., Goodman, R. A., and Bowman, B. A. (2014). "Prevention of chronic disease in the 21st century: elimination of the leading preventable causes of premature death and disability in the USA." *The Lancet*, *384*(9937), 45–52.

Bloch, C. (2016). *Passion and paranoia: Emotions and the culture of emotion in academia*. London and New York: Routledge.

Ellingson, L. L. (2017). *Embodiment in qualitative research*. New York and London: Routledge.

Frank, A. W. (1995). *The wounded storyteller: Body, illness, and ethics*. Chicago: University of Chicago Press.

Geist-Martin, P., Sharf, B., and Yamasaki, J. (Eds.). (2017). *Storied health and illness: Communicating personal, cultural, and political complexities*. Long Grove, IL: Waveland Press.

Goffman, E. (1959). *The presentation of self in everyday life*. Garden City, NY: Doubleday.

Haraway, D. (1988). "Situated knowledges: The science question in feminism and the privilege of partial perspective." *Feminist studies*, *14*, 575–599. doi: 10.2307/3178066

Harter, L. M. (2013). *Imagining new normals: A narrative framework for health communication*. Dubuque, IA: Kendall Hunt.

Mairs, N. (1997). Carnal acts. In K. Conboy, N. Medina, and S. Stanbury (Eds.), *Writing on the body: Female embodiment and feminist theory* (pp. 296–305). New York: Columbia University Press.

Sav, A., King, M. A., Whitty, J. A., Kendall, E., McMillan, S. S., Kelly, F., ... and Wheeler, A. J. (2015). "Burden of treatment for chronic illness: a concept analysis and review of the literature." *Health Expectations*, *18*(3), 312–324.

Sotirin, P. (2010). "Autoethnographic mother-writing: Advocating radical specificity." *Journal of Research Practice*, *6*(1). Article M9. Retrieved from: http://jrp.icaap.org/index.php/jrp/article/view/220/220

Acknowledgments

First, profound gratitude is extended to this volume's contributors. Without your willingness to share your health narratives this volume would not have been possible. Thank you to our colleagues, Penn State Health St. Joseph and other public health advocates who support narrative health. A special thank you to Alexandria Yeager and Jocelyn Vargas for your editorial expertise and critical eye for detail and Corina Pillar for your early research and commitment to health communication scholarship. This book was made possible, in part by the generous support of Dan and Sarah Rothermel.

KESHA MORANT WILLIAMS

Kesha Morant Williams is especially grateful to her *village* for their support during the writing of this book. Special recognition goes out to her husband, Algernon Williams, her children Jackson Alexander, Mitchell Keith, her bonus son Rex Ezra. Sincere gratitude is expressed to her foundation; her parents Willie and Frances Morant and her siblings Willie "Billy" Morant Jr. and Frances "Selena" Morant.

To my husband, Al, thank you for always being in my corner and supporting my dreams in anyway that you can. You are my cheerleader, my promoter, and most importantly my life partner. To my children, I work hard to build a legacy for you. When physicians said highly improbable, you showed us otherwise. Thank you for being my precious gifts from above; you are the best part of me. My parents, Willie and Frances Morant, for teaching me from a very early age the value of hard work and delayed gratification. Also, for keeping your grandchildren entertained so I could focus on this book! To my brother, you have always amazed me by how no matter what you encounter you always find a way to offer me support. And, most important to this project, my sister and co-editor Selena the inspiration behind this collection. I am so grateful for who you are in my life; you make me a better mother, sister, and friend. Thank you for allowing to me co-narrate your experience.

FRANCES SELENA MORANT

Frances “Selena” Morant would like to express extreme gratitude to those family members and friends who have supported her along this journey. Special recognition goes out to her children, Myles Cameron McKinney and Malina Camille McKinney, her parents Willie and Frances Morant, brother Willie J. Morant Jr., and sister, Kesha Morant Williams.

To my children, you have been my biggest motivators, inspiration, and reason for remaining strong throughout my greatest challenges. Myles, I thank you for being my calm, quiet, logical voice during the storm. Malina, I thank you for being my creative, high-energy, comedic relief during the most difficult of times. Thanks for being the best hugger in my life. I love you both to the moon and beyond. We are the power of three. To my parents Willie Sr. and Frances Morant, for lighting the fire to pursue education and to stay strong and positive; regardless of life’s setbacks. I appreciate you being surrogate parents to my children and stepping in to help me raise them to become amazing young adults. To my brother, “Billy” who has always been the biggest supporter of my *dreamchasing*. You have always been my cheerleader, and for that, I am eternally grateful. And lastly, to my sister Kesha for believing in me; even when I didn’t believe in myself. Thank you for being my best friend, my sister, and my inspiration. You have given lupus a greater voice, and most of all you have fostered in me a renewed hope and focus for all of my current and future endeavors. Thank you, my sister. I love you; always and forever.

Introduction

Not an Illusion

Kesha Morant Williams

Once upon a time, there was a group of vibrant, engaging, and productive women diligently working to chart their course in this increasingly complicated society. From recent college graduates to career professionals the women in this collection gain agency by sharing their stories about their experience of living with an invisible illness. Invisible chronic illness entails the traditional characteristics of chronic illness, along with attributes of conditions that are not perceptible, not noticeable, and not evident to others, an illness *unseen* (Vickers, 1998). This book extends this definition by also including examples of how culture, lifestage, and the illness experience can lead to invisibility. Living with an invisible illness can be a frustrating and isolating experience because the undetectable symptoms make it difficult for diagnosis, which often leads to disbelief that the illness exists. Some patients have been accused fabricating or exaggerating their health condition. Patients often feel isolated because they experience their suffering alone (Gallop, et. al, 2012; Vickers, 1998). In addition to isolation, for many people, invisible illness also causes a biography disruption. Biography disruption is the idea that chronic illness affects daily life, individual identity, self-reliance, and personal relationships (Bury, 2008). Illness introduces discontinuity in a person's life trajectory. People living with a chronic illness sometimes have to adjust or recreate their identity. According to Jackson, Glenn, and Morant Williams (2012), people pay particular attention to and think about their identity during times of crisis. Illness complications might require a person to change careers, forgo having children, or renegotiate their educational goals. For many people, the unpredictability of the illness experience disrupts their ability to engage socially. Additionally, many people adjust to a measured lifestyle (Lowe and McBride-Henry, 2012). This newly renegotiated identity leaves people who are living with the invisible illness analyzing what has been lost from their old identity, what remains the same, and what is new?

This book provides a platform that recognizes that "science gives us a way of thinking about disease, but the arts and humanities provide insight, context, and understanding of what it means to be ill. Diseases are black and white, described by facts, figures, categories, and concepts, but illness is coloured, nuanced by context, and shaped by individual circumstances" (Shanahan, 2012, para. 6). While many narratives privilege the biomedical perspective, this volume offers the alternative; a collection of stories based on the non-privileged storyteller. Akin to communication theorist Walter Fisher, the women in this book propose that life is a series of ongoing narratives that are shaped by our histories, culture, and character. This means that our identities are informed by our interaction with society and culture.

In May 2012, I sat in a crowded audience awaiting the unveiling of "Portraits of Hope for Lupus" a traveling art exhibit for lupus awareness at the Capitol Rotunda in Harrisburg, Pennsylvania. The exhibit, twenty portraits composed mostly of women, created a beautiful narrative about the lived experiences of persons diagnosed with the invisible chronic illness, lupus. While my knowledge of lupus had significantly increased since my sister's 2005 diagnosis; I was ignorant to the many ways lupus functions as a chameleon in the human body (CDC, 2017). But as I sat in the audience and viewed each portrait and listened to the accompanying narrative I realized that each experience overflowed with embodied knowledge. As a health communication scholar, I have used my platform to increase awareness about lupus; however, more and more, I find myself engaged in conversation with women living with other invisible illnesses who are actively searching for someone to listen to their story; someone to hear their voice. Creating a space to listen, a space for voice was the catalyst for this book, *Reifying Women's Experiences with Invisible Illness*.

In *The Wounded Storyteller*, Arthur Frank challenges the ideology that seeking medical attention requires that one surrenders their personal narrative and adopt a prescribed medical narrative. Rejecting the notion that a person's story must be secondary to all-knowing health professionals; Frank asserts that health practitioners must incorporate a sociocultural approach to health care, which addresses a broader definition of health and healing (e.g., psyche, identity).

Stories, specifically first-person accounts, create a space to advocate on behalf of the individual who is chronically ill rather than focusing on the perspective of medical professionals. It is empowering for a person to have the resources to tell their own story. Nevertheless, Frank (2012) is quick to point out that storytelling is not about proving a position rather, "people's stories report their reality as they need to tell it, as well as reporting, what they believe their listeners are prepared to hear," (p. 38). Often, the ill person feels obligated to tell their story in a way that pleases their audience's expectation, and responds a certain way even if they don't feel it, or believe it. Storytelling creates an opportunity to "...in the simplest sense gather voices to give them a more evocative voice so that these storytellers can hear each other, and so they can be heard collectively," (p. 36).

Mohan Dutta (2008) advances this position and centers it within cultural health communication scholarship. In *Communicating Health* Dutta argues that culture and context must be considered in any discourse about health. Mainstream western ideology is consistently privileged over that of the ill person in many cultural contexts. According to Dutta, gender and racial inequalities are ever-present examples of power and privilege.

Dutta (2008) writes:

> These positions of the expert and of the research subject are predicated on power; those with access to power get to construct conceptual maps, develop problem configurations, and implement solutions in the target community—a community which typically exists at the margins of the power configurations and hence must serve as the object under investigation. It is important to question this expert-object relationship in the context of the geographic, socio-economic, racial, and gendered lines along which it plays out....[the fact that] a large percentage of services directed towards women are offered by men, demonstrates gender inequalities. (p. 49)

By dismissing sociocultural factors, the full experience of the ill person is silenced as she is told to adopt a prescribed medical narrative. Nigerian writer Chimamanda Ngozi Adichie echoed this point in her groundbreaking speech, *The Danger of a Single Story*. The purpose of this collection is to provide a platform that highlights the health narratives of women. Women, although they live longer than men, research supports that women are more likely to have "chronic debilitating conditions" (Needman and Hill, 2014, p. 1) than men. Also, while there are clear biological differences between males and females, sociocultural issues also impact health outcomes. Further, research supports that societal roles, body image, and medical interactions impact how women respond to and experience health (McDonough, Walters and Strohschein, 2002; Morant Williams, in press).

The chapters in this collection are reflective of narrative inquiry as it is composed of diverse definitions, methodologies, and approaches (Sools, 2012) yet it remains in line with Ochs and Capps (2001) *Living Narrative* as the stories in this book are multidimensional, highly tellable, personal experiences. Through the lens of sisterhood and social support, this book opens with *My Sister's Keeper* a co-constructed narrative about my sister (and co-editor) and myself. In the chapter, I use storytelling and relational ethics, to highlight how Selena and I grappled with a critical health incident she experienced triggered by systemic lupus erythematosus. This chapter examines invisibility, living loss, liminality, and family—and more specifically, social support within the sibling relationship.

In chapter 2, Nicole Defenbaugh creatively uses the theme of a love-story to examine the mind-body connection in treating ulcerative colitis through diet change and counseling. In the chapter, Defenbaugh also unpacks how these practices have helped shape her current state of health. This is a story about the beginning stages of love and a (re)mission where values are explored, perceptions are queried, and the question about whether this identity will last is always foremost in the author's mind.

The next three chapters focus on navigating an invisible illness as an undergraduate student or post-baccalaureate scholar. In "*A Semblance of Normalcy: Social Isolation and the Burden of Looking Well*," Hannah Thyberg explores the topics of illness and isolation. In this chapter, Thyberg highlights how illness and isolation influenced her ability to form and maintain relationships, both as an undergraduate student and presently. Like many first-year college students, the author arrived ready to discover the world and herself. Wide-eyed and open-armed, she set out to embrace her idyllic future. However, just a few weeks into her first semester she began to experience significant health issues and was later diagnosed with fibromyalgia.

Similarly, chapter 4 also focuses on the undergraduate college experience as Emily Pfender reflects on navigating life as a college student suffering from Borderline Personality Disorder. As an honor student and teaching assistant, Pfender argues that she does not fit the stereotypical representation of the mentally ill. Through personal narrative, Pfender examines myths surrounding mental illness and describes how she used transparency and disclosure as a means of gaining the trust and support of professors, coworkers, family, and friends, which aided in her successful matriculation through college.

Chapter 5 chronicles recent college graduate Launick Saint-Fort who was diagnosed with Postural Orthostatic Tachycardia Syndrome (POTS) just a few months into her post-baccalaureate health-related research fellowship. In this chapter, Saint-Fort recounts her plight with the onset of POTS and the difficult road to diagnosis. Furthermore, this chapter introduces the intersections of race, gender, and socioeconomics as the author reflects on her journey as an international woman of color in the United States discovering a new self and career path.

Though vastly different illness experiences, intersections of race, gender, and career are reflected in the chapters that follow. In chapter 6, "*When Lifestage Matters: A Narrative Account of a Pregnancy-Related Invisible Illness*," Eletra S. Gilchrist Petty mixes the analytic with the personal by sharing her experience as a professional woman of color with an invisible illness that only ensues during pregnancy. Through narratives, the author describes how the illness resulted in the miscarriage of her twin daughters five-and-a-half months into the pregnancy and connects the illness experience to mortality, social support, and overall reproductive health and awareness.

In chapter 7, Cerise L. Glenn explores professional identity negotiation as an African American female professor living with the rare invisible chronic illness Hidradenitis Suppurativa. In the chapter, Glenn unpacks aspects of black feminist thought frame (re)learning self-identity and empowerment. Lastly, socio-economic and class privilege is interrogated as part of learning to embrace a "differently" abled lifestyle with an illness that's often invisible to friends, family, and co-workers.

Chapter 8, "*Duty, Honor, Country…Sickness: Finding strength in my quarter century battle with Gulf War Illness*" skillfully examines intersections of race, gender, and career, specifically military service while chronicling the author's solitary sojourn through illnesses and diagnosis. Elizabeth Desnoyers-Colas is a retired senior USAF captain, third generation military, and one of the first women able to serve in a combat zone. This chapter chronicles her bouts of physical and cognitive weakness that have significantly affected and shaped her professional and personal interactions.

Annette Madlock Gatison asks readers to expand their understanding of invisibility and illness in her chapter, "*Complicit in Concealing Illness: Black Women, Beauty, Identity, and Breast Cancer.*" Using African American women and breast cancer as a frame, Madlock Gatison asserts that socially constructed beauty standards implore women to perform healthiness; hence hiding or removing the visual reminders of the illness experience. Additionally, the chapter explores how the trifecta of strength emanating from the rhetoric of breast cancer warrior metaphors, Christian faithtalk, and the strong black woman ideology influenced African American female breast cancer survivor's perceptions of self and how others perceived them.

Closing as it opened, like chapter 1, the final chapter uses a co-constructed narrative linked to sister-friends and social support. Through the lens of breast cancer, chapter author Sun Wei aligns with Madlock Gatison's approach to expanding understanding of invisibility and illness by focusing on how minority invisibility hinders breast cancer survivorship and support for cancer patients in the Chinese American community.

The chapters in this book ask the reader to expand their understanding of disease and illness. Through narrative inquiry the authors in this volume blend the analytic and the personal to share their health narrative but also to support that while the biomedical prospective is an important one, it is not the only one. There is power is allowing a person to tell their own story on their own terms. This collection of stories is an attempt to increase opportunities for embodied knowledge. The more we normalize patient perspectives the more likely we are to move toward *stories* instead of a *story*.

REFERENCES

Adichie, C. N. (2009). The danger of a single story. Retrieved from https://www.ted.com/talks/chimamanda_adichie_the_danger_of_a_single_story

Bury, M. (2008). Chronic illness as biography disruption. *Sociology of Health and Illness*, *4*(2), 167–182. doi: 10.111/1467–9566.ep11339939

Dutta, M. (2008). *Communicating Health: A culture-centered approach*. Malden, MA: Polity.

Frank, A. W. (1995). *The Wounded Storyteller: Body, Illness, and Ethics*. Chicago: University of Chicago Press.

Frank, A. W. (2012). "Practicing Dialogical Narrative Analysis." In *Varieties of Narrative Analysis,* edited by James A. Holstein and Jaber F. Gubrium, 33–52. Thousand Oaks, CA: Sage.

Gallop, K, Nixon, A., Swinburn, P., Sterling, K.L., Naegeli, A.N., Silk, M. E. T. (2012). Development of a conceptual model of health-related quality of life for systemic Lupus erythematosus (SLE) from the patients' perspective. *Lupus, 21*(9), 934–943. dio:10.1177/0961203312441980.

Jackson, R., Glenn, C. and Morant Williams, K. M., (2012). Self Identity. In A. Kurylo (Ed.), *Inter/Cultural Communication: Representation and construction of culture in everyday*. Thousand Oaks, CA: Sage.

Lowe, P. and McBride-Henry, K. (2012). What factors impact upon the quality of life of elderly women with chronic illnesses: Three women's perspectives. *Contemporary Nurse, 41*(1), p. 18–27. doi:10.5172/conu.2012.41.1.18

McDonough, P., Walters, V., and Strohschein, L. (2002). Chronic stress and the social patterning of women's health in Canada. *Social Science & Medicine*, *54*, 767–782.

Morant Williams, K.M. (forthcoming). But you look fine: The impact of family social support on African American women living with lupus. *Howard Journal of Communications,* (TBA).

Needman, B. and Hill, T. (2014). Mental and physical gendered health links. ResearchGate, 1–5. DOI: 10.1002/9781118410868.wbehibs106

Ochs, E. and Capps, L. (2001) *Living Narrative: Creating lives in everyday storytelling.* Cambridge, MA: Harvard University Press.

Sools, A. (2012). Narrative health research: Exploring big and small stories as analytical tools. *Health: An Interdisciplinary Journal for the Social Study of Health, Illness and Medicine*, *17*(1), 93–110. DOI: https://doi.org/10.1177/1363459312447259

University of College Cork, Ireland. (2012). International symposium on the experience of illness at UCC [Press release]. Retrieved from https://www.ucc.ie/en/about/uccnews/archive/2012/fullstory-172579-en.html

Vickers, M. H. (1998, June). Life at Work with "Invisible" Chronic Illness (ICI): A Passage of Trauma- Turbulent, Random, Poignant. *Administrative Theory & Praxis*, *20*(3), 196–204. doi:128.118.244.41

Wellard, S. (1998). Constructions of chronic illness. *Nursing Studies*, *35*, 49–55.

Chapter One

My Sister's Keeper

Sibling Social Support and Chronic Illness

Kesha Morant Williams

I am sitting on my sister's couch right now. I am in her house all alone. I am sleepy but anxious. I want to be at the hospital with her, yet I want to ball up in a corner by myself. My sister is the strongest person I know. She is a single mother, and she is living with an aggressive chronic disease. Her surgery was considered routine. But, nothing is routine with an immune system like my sisters. I love my sister. I will always be my sister's keeper.—KMW

Selena is a beautiful woman in her mid forties. Her sun-kissed skin glows as if she is an inhabitant of a Caribbean island. Her infectious smile brightens the room and her commitment to her children made me yearn for motherhood. To the outside world, she is a strong single mother who has managed to survive a divorce, raise her children, and thrive in her career and educational pursuits; nevertheless, she is also a woman living with an invisible disease.

Lupus is a chronic, autoimmune disease that can damage any part of the body. Unfortunately, it is one of the least recognized diseases and is one of the most difficult diseases to diagnose. A healthy immune system fights off foreign bodies protecting it from viruses, such as the flu as well as harmful bacteria and germs. A person living with lupus has a compromised immune system. In other words, a person's immune system is tricked into believing that healthy tissues are unhealthy tissues or foreign bodies. The body turns against itself and causes significant harm to a person's organs and overall health. Those who are lucky manage their lupus flares with medication and life modifications; those who do not die from lupus-related complications (Lupus, 2016). When a person is living with lupus everything associated with her health is interconnected. Therefore, when my sister had a surgery that within a healthy immune system was considered routine her body went haywire, and she was hospitalized because of complications. Since her 2005 diagnosis, my sister has been hospitalized more times than we can count and has experienced lupus flares, which leave her in extreme pain and immobile. This story is all too common for those living with or supporting someone living with lupus.

Emerging from a cultural studies framework stories can also be used as a means of coping with the changes presented throughout the illness experience. These changes are not only reflected in the life of the ill person but also those closest to her, more specifically her children. In Selena's case, this is demonstrated when she withdraws to hide her physical pain in an attempt to limit her children's exposure to her illness experience. When the pain is too great, she depends on her support system to pick up on her signals and meet both her needs, as well as the needs of her children (White, Mendoza, White, and Bond, 2009). This is sometimes a challenge, particularly if signals are misunderstood. The ambiguous nature of the disease leaves little room for traditional loss markers. This pushes my sister and her loved ones into a liminal space creating considerable confusion about the desired type and timing of support and assistance (Boss and Couden, 2002).

Nevertheless, the permanence of sibling relationships traditionally allows them to endure challenges, such as the impact of a chronic illness, that are likely to destroy voluntary relationships. Many people learn how to provide support in sibling relationships. Siblings turn to each other to fill companionship, comfort, affection, friendship, and intimacy needs. More specific to this study, women are closer to their siblings than men (Goetting, 1986) and are more likely to seek emotional support (Cicirelli, 1995). Sisters become closer during adulthood (Bedford, 1993; Ross and Milgram, 1982) and serve as an increased source of support during periods of loss and times of crisis (Troll, 1975).

METHOD

In this work, relational ethics (Austin, 2008) are employed as my sister and I allow the outside world to peek into our lived experiences. Relational ethics are particularly important in autoethnographies because by using personal experiences both the autoethnographer and those related to the experience are implicated. Also, there are often interpersonal connections between the autoethnographer and other participants; therefore the consideration of relational ethics is essential.

Ellis, Adams, and Bochner (2011) further explicate by writing:

> Autoethnographers thus consider "relational concerns" as a crucial dimension of inquiry (Ellis, 2007, p. 25; Trahar, 2009) that must be kept uppermost in their minds throughout the research and writing process. On many occasions, this obligates autoethnographers to show their work to others implicated in or by their texts, allowing these others to respond, and/or acknowledging how these others feel about what is being written about them and allowing them to talk back to how they have been represented in the text. (para. 30)

Through my sister's stories and mine, I use qualitative inquiry to unpack a critical incident along my sister's journey with lupus. Using collaborative elements of autoethnography and narrative inquiry this piece explores sibling social support and chronic illness. Autoethnography is defined as an "autobiographical genre of writing and research that displays multiple layers of consciousness, connecting the personal to the cultural" (Ellis and Bochner, 2000, p. 739). According to Ellis and Bochner (2006), an autoethnographer is "first and foremost a communicator and a storyteller" (p. 111); therefore, autoethnography uses the telling of stories as a method for obtaining and interpreting data directly linked to the lived experience of the participant, in this case, my sister and me. The overt inclusion of personal experience is a unique characteristic of this approach, making it particularly relevant to use when exploring a person's illness narrative.

Many scholars evaluate the goodness of autoethnographies by using criteria based on Laurel Richardson's (2000) foundational piece *Evaluating Ethnography.* This criterion includes substantive contribution, aesthetic merit, reflexivity, impact, and expresses a reality. While there is considerable resistance to linking evaluative methods to the practice of autoethnography, I found it an appropriate addition to this piece as these characteristics strengthen the framework of this autoethnographic work, which contributes to our cultural understanding of the illness experience rather than solely focusing on the physical impact of a disease. The effectiveness of the criteria is measured by the audience's response (ability to connect with research, ability to move toward some change) to the work (Ellis et al., 2011). Storytelling creates a powerful opportunity to establish a connection between the autoethnographer and the listener as a story never solely belongs to its teller. Arthur Frank (2012) asserts that there is value in "hearing how multiple voices find expression within any single voice. A storyteller tells a story that is his or her own, but no story is ever entirely anyone's own. Stories are composed of fragments of previous stories, artfully rearranged but never original" (Frank, 2012, p. 35). Narrative as text, one of the most common uses of narrative, is used to share my sister's stories. "Bruner's (1986) widely accepted definition of a narrative mode of thinking as engagement in sequential, action-oriented, detail-driven thought. Central to the narrative mode is attention to the uniqueness of human storytellers as existential beings, capable of reflecting on their lives and of striving for something" (Sools, 2013, p. 94). This piece expands the body of literature on social support but more specifically it creates linkages between sibling social support and chronic illness.

THE JOURNEY

Living Loss

When linked with illness the term loss is most often referring to end of a life; however, the connection between illness and loss is much broader than this basic framework. Kelly (2008) uses the term living loss and asserts that "loss is alive and embodies not only as an emotional but also a corporeal experience that is ongoing and changing" (p. 338). Living loss explains the experiences the chronically ill person (i.e., Selena) encounters. It also links the sociocultural framework that organizes the way loss narratives are created, shared, and interpreted. Living loss navigates the tension between the sociocultural framework and the experiences of the individuals being affected by loss.

Selena views her experience with lupus as an evolutionary process. Her stories highlight the continuous change she experienced before and during her diagnosis. When thinking back on early signs and symptoms, she felt physically fatigue and achy and experienced brain fog. In the years leading to her diagnosis, she suffered with increased and more substantial health changes. When reflecting back, she recognizes lupus symptoms she experienced more than twenty years ago.

> I can trace a lot of symptoms back to 1990 when I was in college and in 1998 when I was in the Army. Headaches, pleurisy (I was rushed to the hospital, felt like a heart attack). When my son was about learning how to ride a bike, I was running behind him holding the bike. Later that day and several days afterward, I was so sore and felt like I had pulled several muscles. I couldn't understand why it felt like every muscle in every part my body. I couldn't walk or do much of anything and felt like I was out of shape. Fast forward several years, I now realize that I had sent my body into a spinning lupus flare!

Since 2005, she has been diagnosed with Systematic Lupus Erthematosus, Sjogren's Syndrome, and Raynaud's Disease. In addition, her compromised immune system leaves her vulnerable to infection and extended recuperation periods. However, her evolutionary process is not limited to her physical health. In line with the literature on the mental health effects of chronic illness, my sister sometimes lives a life of isolation as she copes with flares and other lupus related challenges. She constantly strives to embrace her new normal yet at times is overcome with feelings of sadness, frustration, or anger. Also, current research supports that clinical depression may be linked to lupus medications (Gallop et al., 2012; Lupus and Depression, 2016).

Living loss also affects her interpersonal social health as it forces her to renegotiate the quality of her relationships with friends, family, and others with whom she is in contact. The quantity and quality of one's social relationships have both long and short-term effects on one's mental and physical health as well as overall health behavior (Cornwell and Waite, 2008). The effects of the disease shifts her ability to engage with others as she did prior to her diagnosis. At times she views the disease as baggage that others may not be interested in carrying. For example, she asserts:

> Honestly, it has kept me from forming, developing and maintaining relationships. Despite dating and spending time with an individual, the effort and work to keep this going are minimal because, in the back of my mind, I wonder if a man would willingly sign-up for the challenges that come with chronic illness. It's a barrier to being open and honest because of hiding this part of myself.

This passage is also representative of living loss as a reflection of liminality. Turner (1969) described liminality as a middle space "neither here nor there; they are betwixt and between the positions assigned and arrayed by law, custom, convention, and ceremony" (p. 95). Kelly (2008) continues that liminality can be a troubling experience because "…there is no sociocultural classification or a medical diagnosis of where 'there' is…" (p. 336). The term dates back as far as 1884, was introduced to anthropology by Arnold Van Gennep (1909), but did not gain popularity until Turner (1969) borrowed and expanded upon Van Gennep's work. More recently, scholars described liminality as a phase in an illness episode and have researched its place in cancer patients (Little, Jordens, Montgomery, and Philipson, 1998) as well as HIV/AIDs patients and caregivers (Kelly, 2008). Similarly, this research extends this description by connecting liminality, lupus, and living loss.

A person living with lupus functions within a liminal space because as with other chronic illnesses, there is no cure. Lupus is described as a chameleon disease because it manifests itself and can affect those living with the illness in completely different ways. Periods of wellness can last years; however, even during these periods, Selena is very conscious of the choices she makes and how they might affect her health. In other words, even in times of wellness, she still lives in liminality. Lupus complications might require a person to change careers, forego having children or renegotiate her educational goals. The disease disrupts a person's ability to function socially or to engage in activities. The unpredictability of the disease forces many patients to adjust to a slower pace of life. Other patients assert that when they are in remission, they accomplish a great deal because they cannot when flares arise (Lowe and McBride-Henry, 2012). Over time, Selena learned what triggers set off flares and has grown accustomed to avoiding these foods, products, or activities.

This unpredictability makes it difficult for Selena to maintain employment or pursue her doctorate; thus, she finds herself living in limbo. For example, she earned a bachelor of science in psychology, served in the Army, completed nursing school, and maintained an active social life. Shortly after beginning her nursing career, she became ill and was later diagnosed with lupus. Her immune system was compromised and could not handle the environmental conditions of her new career. Hence, just a few short months after completing nursing school and beginning her new position she was pushed into a holding pattern. She later returned to graduate school and earned a master of science in counseling and yet again, began a new career. Yet again, the lupus flares begin, and she cannot maintain her client load and shifts from full-time to part-time, to a medical leave of absence. She began working toward her doctoral degree but finds that brain fog limits her ability to concentrate in a rigorous program. She again finds herself stuck in a holding pattern—*neither here nor there*.

Relationship

Selena and I are not only sisters—we are friends. Five years my senior, she helped me navigate my transition from high school to college. She listened intently when I asked her about everything from birth control to sorority life. She never judged me but always told me to be safe and make wise decisions. When she was pregnant with my nephew, she lived in Virginia. I went to stay with her a few weeks before and after his birth. We did a practice drive to the hospital so that I would be prepared to take her. But when her water broke in the Target parking lot my mind went blank, and I had no idea where I was going. She told me to take her to a friend's apartment. We had purchased a frozen pizza, and she wanted to eat before she went to the hospital. She kneeled on the floor on her hands and knees and breathed through the contractions. Eventually, she gave up on the pizza, and we left for the hospital. A few hours after Myles was born she asked: "Did they eat my pizza?" My sister has a quiet spirit, is slow to anger and will find peace in the most challenging situations. Her ability to thrive and live life on purpose gives me strength when dealing with my own challenges. Although there are any number of incidents (Bitner, Booms, and Mohr, 1990) that can articulate the bond my sister and I share, in the section that follows, I describe one experience as my sister's caretaker shortly after a routine surgery.

An incident is defined as an observable human activity that is complete enough to allow is an event outside the range of normal experience that is sudden, unusual, and unexpected, disrupts one's sense of control, involves the perception of a threat to life and may include elements of physical or emotional loss. These incidents have the power to overwhelm the coping abilities of an individual. Also, the incident must make a significant contribution, either positively or negatively, to an event or phenomenon (Bitner et al., 2011). This critical health incident is reflected by my narrative description of the experience.

Today I *finally* cried.

I walked in my house and straight up the stairs to run my bath water. When I am stressed, overwhelmed or want a break from reality I run a hot bubble bath, pour a glass of wine, turn on some music, and soak it all away. I just returned home from my extended stay with my sister. Her surgery was the week before spring break. Her couch became my bed. My niece and nephew, (Myles and Malina affectionately referred to as M&M) became my responsibility. I wrote a note to excuse my nephew from school on the day of my sister's surgery and another note to release him early from school for his orthodontist appointment. I helped my homeschooled niece with most of her school assignments, recruited my nephew to help her with math and tried to remember if she had band or orchestra practice each morning. I drove them to school, church, art class, my parents' house, and to visit their mom in the hospital. I gained an even higher level of respect for my sister. She did all of this running, maintained a job, and managed a chronic illness —*with a smile*. After a week I had stopped combing my hair, wore the same sweat pants three times, and forgot to eat a few meals. Yet as I sat my tub with tears streaming down my face I was quickly reminded that running errands and maintaining order was the easy part. The part that causes me such angst, which keeps me awake at night, is this space of liminality. Even though I had returned home to my *normal* life, my sister was still in the hospital being poked and probed with no answers in sight. I leaned my tablet against the counter and turned on Pandora and used a jar of Vaseline to position my cell phone screen toward the bathtub just in case my sister called or texted, everyone else will have to wait.

As I close my eyes, the images from Tuesday morning filled my mind. My sleepy niece sat on the edge of her bed ready for band practice. I walked down the hall to my sister's room, but she was not there. My heart rate increased as I walked into the dark bathroom. There she sat shaking uncontrollably. Her teeth chattered so badly I could barely understand her words. Was she having a seizure? Was she having a stroke? I was her caretaker, but I did not know what to do. *"Cold. I'm cold"* was all I could understand. I wrap her in her robe and hug her tightly. The shaking stops but, she is exhausted and weak. I have seen my sister in pain many times but never this, never a loss of control. Though I tried to hide it, I was terrified. I help her back to bed. She breathed deeply and said she would be fine while I took her children to school. I do not want to leave, but I do not want to scare or disrupt their lives any more than necessary. I pick up her phone and text a friend. "Can you come over here? The kids have school and an orthodontist appointment. Selena can't be by herself today. Please call or text me on my phone."

I convince myself that she would be fine for the hour I would be gone and I would find someone to come over when I take M&M to their appointment. My niece and nephew get into my car full of energy and chatter. They make jokes about something they watched on television and giggle uncontrollably. I, on the other hand, struggled to keep my watery eyes from overflowing onto my face. I rubbed my eyes, instead of wiping them and adjust my glasses. Perhaps my actions will serve as a manageable disguise. It does not. The car falls silent. They each stare out the window the rest of the drive. I drop my niece off at the middle school for band practice. She gets out in silence and shuts the door. I drive my nephew down the street to his high school and manage to ask him if he needed lunch money? I offer a weak smile and tell him to have a good day. I drive back to middle school and wait for Malina to finish her practice. When I am alone, I chat on the phone with my mom and a friend. I express my concern and that I want to take Selena to the hospital. My other line beeps. I answer the call and hear my sister-friend's voice. "Kesha, Selena isn't good. I'm on my way to her house, but you have the keys, and she can't get downstairs." I run through the middle school in a panic searching for the band room. My niece was sitting on the right side of the stage in the clarinet section. I motion for her to leave and mouth emergency to the band teacher. He nods his head and Malina runs out of the school behind me.

"Is it mommy?" asks my niece.

"Yes, she needs us now," I responded.

I yell at drivers, red lights, and stop signs as I rush to get back to her house. Malina yells too. She runs in the house to check on her mom as I park the car. A few minutes later my brother and, a few sister-friends arrive. We get my sister to the hospital and into triage. Her fever is high enough to cause febrile seizures. Exactly a week after a routine surgery she was back in the hospital with an infection in her body and her blood. The nurses worked for two hours to find a viable vein to insert her IV. With each attempt Selena's face wenches a bit more—eventually she begins to scream. The nurses admit defeat and contact an anesthesiologist who finally starts the IV and begins treatment. I sit in the corner of the room with my sister fielding calls, sending text messages, and helping her answer questions. Through her pain, the mother in her does not subside. "The kids need to go to the orthodontist," she said. I want to cancel the appointment and focus on her but the mother in her takes over and, she insists. "They need to go, and they can't be late," I call my brother in the waiting room; he works it out; they make it to their appointment.

Although we knew M&M were nervous and deeply concerned about their mother's health, Selena was determined to keep their lives as *normal* as possible. It was her attempt to protect her *cubs* from her illness as much as possible. Her ex-husband had chosen not to be a part of their lives shortly after he and Selena divorced. Myles was a toddler, and Malina was still in diapers and were too young to have any memories of their father. They know he is alive, he is in the military, and that their parents were once married. I do my best to be a good aunt, and my parents serve as a constant support. They understand their mom's illness. They know that sometimes she is very tired and in pain and that sometimes her migraines are so intense they have to leave her bedroom light off and whisper when speaking. But they also know that there is no co-parent to carry the load or to assure them that their mother will *yet again* pull through this health episode.

They readmit Selena to the hospital; I sit with her most of the evening then leave to help M&M prepare for the next morning. I walk in the house and tell them to start preparing for bed and to gather everything they needed for the next day. The air is heavy. We are trying to keep moving but, we are stuck in liminality. I want to fix it. I want to make their mother better. I want to take the fear and sadness out of their eyes. I know I cannot; they know I cannot. Her health episodes have concerned me in the past, but they have never scared me. I am scared, and they know it. Instead of talking we stand in the hallway outside the bathroom, hold hands and pray. I hug them tight. We go to sleep. The cycle of work for me, school for my niece and nephew, homework, meals, hospital, and bed quickly became routine; but the angst of when will she get better did not. My nephew played video games, my niece sketched in her drawing pad, and I wrote. We each had our way of escaping the uncertainty surrounding her health and what would happen next.

After about two weeks of treatment, procedures that typically worked in forty-eight hours on patients with healthy immune systems had no positive effect on my sister's condition. Instead, it worsened her condition. In addition to the infection and fever, the medicine led to rashes covering her entire body and sores inside her mouth and on her lips. Her medical team is baffled. She is a medical anomaly. It seems that their training in specialized areas has left them incapable of looking at the holistic picture. She is a woman living with an invisible disease that affects her body in ways her medical team cannot seem to understand. Infection specialists and her primary physicians battled over preferred treatments while Selena sat in limbo. Against her primary physicians' suggestions, she sided with the infection specialists and elected to undergo a second major surgery. In recovery, her physician tells her they opened her up but did not find anything. The physician admits that it was likely a lupus flare and had passed on its own; implying that the second surgery was unnecessary—*but who really knows with this chameleon disease*. The recovery from two major abdominal surgeries in under a month is lengthy, to say the least. It appears that this incident is nearing its end and my sister will *yet again* pull through this health episode and return to *normalcy*. The challenge of chronic illness is that it is chronic—it does not go away. It hides, it lurks, it rests, but it is still there teetering on the edge—leaving my sister and her support system in a space of liminality—*neither here nor there.*

A sister is a forever friend.—Author Unknown

Although our sibling relationship is involuntary, our friendship is voluntary. My sister is one of my closest and most trusted friends. The relationship we share includes a blending of characteristics found in both sibling relationships and friendships. Literature supports that except in cases of death, sibling relationships usually last longer than any other relationship a person experiences. When I reflect on my dominant lived experiences my sister was always present—from my first steps to my wedding day, my sister was by my side. As a child she was my guide, and I was her shadow. We learned early in life that sisters looked after each other and were concerned about each other's well-being. As adults, our supportive behaviors extend beyond family obligations. While I must admit, I often feel helpless in this liminal space our random phone conversations and late night sessions of text messaging foster a deeper level of connectivity in our relationship. Our expression of social support is built upon a lifetime of love and commitment.

Friends may come and go, but my sister will always be my sister. Thus in 2005 when she was diagnosed with a disease that I knew nothing about I began to ask her questions and search online for additional clarity. Instead of becoming burdened by her diagnosis my sister became an advocate. She handed out lupus bracelets, pins and discussed the disease among friends and family. I was honored to be in the audience when she was featured in "Portraits of Hope for Lupus: A Traveling Exhibit for Lupus Awareness" I was honored to stand with her as her portrait was formally introduced. My sister's loss narratives suggest that living with a chronic illness can be a lonely place. The effects of lupus have forced her to renegotiate her life script and adjust to living in liminality. There is no such thing as a *normal* day; because even during periods of wellness she is cognizant of the never ending liminality. Since her diagnosis, I have learned how to support Selena during times of illness. In some instances that means texting instead of calling her or when I am in town, washing dishes, folding a load of laundry, or dropping off my niece and nephew wherever they need to be. In other instances it may be listening to her stories, affirming that her frustrations are legitimate and that although I cannot take it away—I am here with her *in this middle place*.

REFERENCES

Austin, W. J. (2008). "Relational ethics." In L. M. Give (Ed.), *The SAGE encyclopedia of qualitative research methods* (pp. 749–50). Thousand Oaks, CA: SAGE Publications. http://dx.doi.org/10.4135/9781412963909.n378

Bedford, V. H. (1993). "Relationships between adult siblings." In A. E. Auhagen and M. von Salisch (Eds.), *Interpersonal relationships* (pp. 119–141). Gottingen, Germany: Hogrefe, Verlage fur Psychologie.

Bitner, M. J., Booms, B. H., and Mohr, L. A. (1990). "The service encounter: Diagnosing favorable and unfavorable incidents." *Journal of Marketing, 54*, 71–84. http://dx.doi.org/10.2307/1252174

Boss, P., and Couden, B. A. (2002). "Ambiguous loss from chronic physical illness: Clinical interventions with individuals, couples, and families." *Journal of Clinical Psychology, 58*(11), 1351–1360. http://dx.doi.org/10.1002/jclp.10083

Cicirelli, V. G. (1995). *Sibling relationships across the lifespan*. New York, NY: Plenum Press.

Cornwell, E. Y., and Waite, L. J. (2008). "Social disconnectedness, perceived isolation, and health among older adults." *Journal of Health and Social Behaviors, 50*(1), 31–48. http://dx.doi.org/10.1177/002214650905000103

Ellis, C., and Bochner, A. P. (2000). "Autoethnography, personal narrative, reflexivity." In N. K. Denzin & Y. S. Lincoln (Eds.), *Handbook of qualitative research* (2nd ed.). (pp. 733–768). Thousand Oaks, CA: Sage.

Ellis, C., and Bochner, A. P. (2006). "Analyzing analytic autoethnography: An autopsy." *Journal of Contemporary Ethnography, 35*(4), 429–449. http://dx.doi.org/10.1177/0891241606286979

Ellis, C., Adams, T. E., and Bochner, A. P. (2011). "Autoethnography: An overview." *Forum: Qualitative Social Research, 12*(1). http://www.qualitative-research.net/index.php/fqs/article/view/1589/3095

Frank, A. W. (2012). "Practicing dialogical narrative analysis." In J. A. Holstein and J. F. Gubrium (Eds.), *Varieties of Narrative Analysis* (pp. 33–52). Thousand Oaks, CA: Sage.

Gallop, K., Nixon, A., Swinburn, P., Sterling K., Naegeli, A., Silk, M. E. (2012). "Development of a conceptual model of health-related quality of life for Systemic Lupus Erythematosus (SLE) from the patient's perspective." *Lupus, 21*(9), 934–43. http://dx.doi.org/10.1177/0961203312441980

Goetting, A. (1986). "The developmental task of siblingship over the lifecycle." *Journal of Marriage and Family, 48*(4), 703–714. http://dx.doi.org/10.2307/352563

Grossberg, L., Cary, N., and Treichler, P. (1992). *Cultural studies*. New York, NY: Routledge.

Kelly, A. (2008). "Living loss: An exploration of the internal space of liminality." *Mortality, 13*(4), 335–350. http://dx.doi.org/10.1080/13576270802383915

Little, M., Jordens, C. F. C., Paul, K., Montgomery, K., and Philipson, B. (1998). "Liminality: A major category of the experience of cancer illness." *Social Science Medicine, 47*(10), 1485–1494. http://dx.doi.org/10.1016/S0277–9536(98)00248-

Lowe, P., and McBride-Henry, K. (2012). "What factors impact upon the quality of life of elderly women with chronic illnesses: Three women's perspectives." *Contemporary Nurse, 41*(1), 18–27. http://dx.doi.org/10.5172/conu.2012.41.1.18

Lupus. (2016). *Center for Disease Control and Prevention*. Retrieved from http://www.cdc.gov/lupus

Lupus and Depression. (2016). *Lupus Foundation of America*. Retrieved from http://www.lupus.org/depression

Richardson, L. 2000. "Evaluating ethnography." *Qualitative Inquiry, 6*(2), 253–255. http://dx.doi.org/10.1177/107780040000600207

Ross, H. G., and Milgram, J. I. (1982). "Important variables in adult sibling relationships. A qualitative study." In M. E. Lamb and B. Sutton-Smith (Eds.), *Sibling relationships: Their nature and significance across the lifespan* (pp. 225–249). Hillsdale, NJ: Lawrence Erlbaum Associates.

Sools, A. (2013). "Narrative health research: Exploring big and small stories as analytical tools." *Health, 17(*1), 93–110. http://dx.doi.org/10.1177/1363459312447259

Troll, L. E. (1975). *Early and middle adulthood: The best is yet to be—maybe*. Monterey, CA: Brooks/Cole Pub. Co.

Turner, V. (1969). *The ritual process: Structure and antistructure*. Chicago, IL: Transaction Publishers.

White, C. P., Mendoza, J., White, M. B., and Bond, C. (2009). "Chronically ill mothers experiencing pain: Relational coping strategies used while parenting young children." *Chronic Illness, 5*, 33–45. http://dx.doi.org/10.1177/1742395309102820

Chapter Two

Temporal Reflections of UC Remission

An Autoethnography of Body Image and Acceptance

Nicole Defenbaugh

My 5'4" nakedness is reflected in the mirrors around me. As I stand before the closet doors where the six panels of mirrors are located, I see myself, my true self, and the reality of my present state of being. I grab my abdomen out of habit—as I have often done since my colon became a source of sickness—and stare at its shape. Unlike the days of my active ulcerative colitis (UC) where my belly was deflated from nutrients and empty of its contents, my abdomen stands full, shapely, filling up the space around it and not apologizing. This is the healthy state I have been waiting for since I was diagnosed; the unimagined dream I dared believe was possible. This is it! I am finally in a state of remission, "the period during which the symptoms of a disease abate or subside" (Wikipedia, 2005, *Remission in Medicine*). I shake my head in disbelief. I am torn between feeling healthy and looking "healthy." The shape of my healthy body is still unfamiliar to me. I do not recognize my own curves as my eyes gaze toward my middle and my fingers grab the skin around my waist in close examination. This body is foreign, bizarre, and abnormal from years of chronic illness. As the days pass into months and months into years since my UC was active, I continue to believe that I will return to my thinner, ill self. Although I never liked my body during times of extreme thinness (figure 2.1), I associated it as part of my chronic identity. Thin is who I was, what I knew, and what I trusted about my body. Weight gain is not the "norm" with Inflammatory Bowel Disease (IBD); a disease in which one's intestinal tract is chronically sick. When an individual with this disease begins to gain weight, and it is not due to the side effects of a medication, such as prednisone, it is likely due to remission. I let go of my abdomen, turn away from the mirrors, and vow not to look in the mirror again…at least not until tomorrow.

This is the first chapter in a love story. A story about finding acceptance and self-love. This is where my illness journey has taken me, on another mission of identity transformation. This is supposed to be a love story about how I have learned to love my "body in remission." I envisioned this story would end with acceptance and forgiveness of myself and what my body has become on this new, yet repeated mission of self-exploration. This new mission of rediscovery has led me down an unknown path of accepting a body that is foreign to me as a chronically ill person. Instead of a classic love story, this is a story about finding myself and seeing myself in a new light with different dimensions. This is a story about the beginning stages of love and a (re)mission where values are explored, perceptions are queried, and the uncertainty about whether this new identity will last is always foremost on my mind.

BACKGROUND

Ulcerative colitis (UC), a common form of Inflammatory Bowel Disease (IBD), remains primarily hidden because active signs of illness are predominantly internal; they occur inside of the colon or other parts of the intestinal tract. The illness may become more visible, for example, after surgical procedures to create an ostomy or ileal pouch-anal anastomosis (IPAA) or j-pouch. J-pouch is named because of the "J" shape created by the small intestine (UCSF Medical Center, 2016). For many who live with IBD, the illness may never feel truly *in*visible because the nature of the disease makes bodily functions more visible. Frequent bathroom visits, pale or clammy skin, excessive weight loss, and uncontrollable bodily noises (e.g., flatulence) can make an internal illness suddenly more visible to others.

The topic of body image and dissatisfaction is not new (Thompson and Stice, 2001), nor is the topic of female body image and chronic illness or disability (Howes, Edwards, and Benton, 2005; White, 2000). Research on IBD and body image has been ongoing for decades. In the late 1980s, individuals with IBD who underwent surgery were surveyed to understand how energy and body image impacted their quality of life (Drossman, Patrick, Mitchell, Zagami, and Appelbaum, 1989). More recently, research has examined quality of life for people with IBD post-surgery (Muller, Prosser, Bampton, Mountifield and Andrews, 2010; da Silva, Hull, Roberts, Ruiz, Wexner, Weiss et al., 2008), or after an IPAA (Larson, Davies, Dozois, Cima, Piotrowicz, Anderson, et al, 2008) to better understand patient perceptions, sexual function, relationships, and body image. Even without surgery, individuals with IBD are concerned about body image (De Rooy, Toner, Maunder, Greenberg, Baron, Steinhart, et al., 2001) and the impact perceptions of IBD have on psychological, social and sexual health (Knowles, Gass and Macrae, 2013). Like many other invisible illnesses, although the illness itself is not apparent to others, the impact of the disease on one's physical, social, and mental well-being can have long-term effects on self-perception and how we think of our bodies and the self-schema we construct (Altabe and Thompson, 1996; Gallagher, 1986). In other words, socially invisible illnesses are highly visible to the person living with the disease. We may be able to hide or "pass" our bodies off as normal to the outside world, but we cannot hide our bodies from ourselves. IBD is not invisible to the person living with it. I argue, one's invisible illness becomes *more* visible to the self over time, blurring the boundary between visibility and invisibility.

I am a chronically ill person. My identity is that of a person with a chronic illness. After fourteen years of being aware of my ill body and its unique needs (i.e., medication, additional vitamins and nutrients), I have internalized both the social gaze and stigmatization often attributed to a visible illness. As Goffman (1963) states, "He [the stigmatized] thus is reduced in our minds from a whole and usual person to a tainted, discounted one" (ibid, 3). In the media we frequently read about stigmatized bodies related to a person's size or shape leading to body-size stigma and stigma attributes (Anderson and Bresnahan, 2013). But stigma also occurs with "injured bodies, and differently acting bodies…" and as a result, "the stigma itself can have a negative effect on a person's well-being and sense of self" (Davis and Quinlan, 2017, p. 201). The internalized stigmatization becomes the norm and thus, the socially invisible illness is highly visible to the ill person. Although this book is about women living with an invisible illness, the illness is not invisible to herself once a person's state of being changes. Over time it becomes difficult, if not impossible, to see one's illness as invisible when multiple medications, diet changes, and "abnormal" bodily functions become the new norm. Normal is a desired state in medicine, a term used frequently by physicians when describing symptoms and identifying patients (Gutzmer and Beach, 2015). The abnormal body *is* the diseased body and normalcy ceases to be seen by the self. And so, even in my current state of remission, I am still an abnormal body living in a state of constant dis-ease with myself. I do not know if my ill identity is coming or going.

METHOD

What better way to understand invisible illness than by writing about one's self (Richards, 2008) from inside the ill person's mind, body, and experiences.

> ...autoethnography is particularly suited to writing about illness and disability. After all, in the end, the lived experience of illness and disability is their reality and those who must live with this reality are those who live it, not those who study it from a distance. (Richards, 2008, p. 1720)

Yamasaki (2017) emphasizes the importance of knowing the patient's experience to further our understanding of health communication, claiming that "we need to elicit and learn from individuals' personal experiences (e.g., pain quality of life, and emotional concerns) and the words they use to speak of wellness, illness, and healing" (p. 3). The stories from the chronically ill help us to better understand the culture of medicine, illness, and health. We learn about their daily experiences and the amount of time spent inside of medical walls, their conversations with colleagues and relationships with loved ones, and their perceptions of self that illuminate normative beliefs and behaviors about the culture of health and illness. As Chang (2008) notes, "the view of culture inside people's mind helps people see themselves as active agents of culture" (p. 21). For others in remission who live in a liminal state of neither long-term health nor chronic illness, we know even less about the impact of remission on the person who was previously ill—since one cannot be in remission without having first been ill. So what is it like for a previously ill-identified person to transition to a state of temporary or permanent health? Since the outcome of this state is unknown, there is much to learn about remission and how this stage impacts an individual's identity. By embarking on an autoethnographic journey I attempt to bridge my past, present, and future selves to understand this new, and unfamiliar state. As Lockford notes, "bridges convey us from where we are to where we want to be" (Lockford, 2014, p. 284). It is on the remission bridge where I stand looking back at my former ill self, exploring my unfamiliar current state, and gazing ahead to the other side of chronic health, all the while uncertain of which direction I'm heading. My body never knows.

BODY

Past: Illness Identity and Digesting Control through Medication and Diet

UC Accountant

I look at the clock on the wall. The short hand paused on 5:00. The time I used to take my afternoon dose of medication, when I would pop another pill, or two, or three. I would then switch my bracelet from my left wrist to my right to signal I had taken my dose (Defenbaugh, 2011, p. 21). At the peak of my illness I took three pills, three times daily; nine pills a day. I increased my literacy skills and now have a higher self-efficacy in managing my health (Chen and Feeley, 2014). The counting, measuring, and problem-solving I did with pills and other health-related behaviors would blow the average healthy person's mind. The next dose I take today, however, won't be until I go to bed in another five to six hours. It is hard to break this old habit, especially one tied to my perception of health. I turn my gaze away from the clock and return my focus on a Netflix episode of *West Wing*.

After fourteen years, I have become quite good at being my own UC accountant. However, I am slowly putting myself out of a job. I am down to taking one pill, two times a day to maintain my state of remission. When I shared this information with my former gastroenterologist, he paused and looked at me inquisitively. I knew what he was going to say next. "That's a good maintenance dose. You really shouldn't go below that…you will always have to take at least one pill for the rest of your life." His words were not news to me. I received the same speech years earlier from another gastroenterologist. What I don't understand, however, is how I can be in remission from UC but still have to take daily medication. This means that according to the medical community, my identity as a chronically ill person never ends. Since I was diagnosed with UC, I will always *have* UC and must take at least one pill a day for life—according to my gastroenterologist. I will need to continue ingesting anti-inflammatory medications to remain in remission. It seems quite confusing to be declared in remission, yet taking pills daily. Common sense would conclude that taking daily medications means that I am *not* in remission and my illness is still active. The common response I have received from clinicians is that my illness is "under control"; whether this means I am officially in remission, remains unknown. The line between active illness and remission in UC, according to the medical community, is blurry. "I am 'betwixt and between' (Turner, 1985) cultures and identities" (Defenbaugh, 2011, p. 136). In the eyes of healthcare, I am chronically ill. My body says otherwise. My body remembers what active UC feels like and looks like. My body remembers the repeated trips to the bathroom, my immune system's response (e.g., skin rashes), and the inability to keep weight on. Now weighted by my own skin with memories of active UC in the past, I feel like I am in a state of remission. The symptoms have abated, and I am attempting to keep it that way by taking a maintenance dose. Every time I pop a pill, however, I still question whether I am truly in remission. I guess it depends on who you ask.

At 10:30 p.m. I head up to bed and walk straight to the bathroom. I have one bottle of pills to treat my inactive UC. ONE bottle. ONE pill. I grab the large, one-month supply of sixty pills, unscrew the childproof cap, and tip the bottle so that one solitary pill falls into my palm. As I do so, three pills spill out. How ironic. It's as if fate is reminding me of the amount I used to take during my active UC. I pick up the extra two pills and put them back into the bottle. I smile, slightly, feeling happy about this maintenance does and simultaneously annoyed because, as the gastroenterologist said, I will never be able to stop taking medications. In this moment, I am acutely aware that I am still a chronically ill person. I have never stopped believing that I can return to a state of healthy "normalcy." As I pop the pill in my hand and chase it with a glass of water, I realize I must have a strong internal locus of control (du Pré, p. 202), a belief that I can control my own destiny, or in this case, my own health/illness. Perhaps internalized from Western doctors since childhood, I have grown to believe that controlling my body (i.e., taking Tylenol for a headache) will result in improved health. This is what I have come to know. If you aren't in control of when you take your meds, you risk a body and illness that is out of control. You risk a crisis. If you change your lifestyle and habits, you might be able to control your illness and return to intermittent health. I have gained control of my health—or sense of healthiness—by controlling what I do to my body. I believe long-term remission is possible if I continue to control what goes in and measure what comes out. This approach has worked in the past and I am currently in a state of pseudo-remission—depending on who you ask.

It's a bit of a mind game convincing your body that it doesn't need any more pills to maintain its health; convincing yourself that everything is okay and that you're not sick. In my mind, no pills equals less control and possible relapse to active UC. Taking pills helps convince me I am in control of my illness. I will continue to take my meds, religiously, like a faithful chronic ill follower. One pill. Two times a day. Check.

Present: Body Image, Self-Discrepancy, and Temporal Comparison

So how does someone shift her identity after fourteen years? Does it have to shift? Does a change in one's appearance demand a shift in one's self-perception? After two years, my health has changed along with my body. My body shape and size have changed, perhaps not dramatically to an onlooker, but significantly to myself; the one who lives inside this body. I regularly examine my body's features for signs of change due to impending illness.

Part I: Mirrored Reflections—Body Image and Temporal Comparison

I have always loved taking a shower. The feeling of the water cascading over my face, across my shoulders and hurtling down to the shower floor. "I'll see you in twenty minutes," I announce to my partner. "See you when you get out," he says with a smile on his face, knowing the typical length of my showers.

I quickly take off my shirt and pants throwing them to the floor, then turn on the water. I reach in to feel the water's icy temperature, knowing it will take a few minutes to warm up, even on this brutally hot summer day. There are mirrors all around my bedroom and bathroom. Three panels on each side of the double closets and three panels in the bathroom. I turn on the fan and switch the dimmer light up ever-so slightly. The rushing water from the shower beckons me to come in, but I stand there, naked, in front of the mirror. I stare and look in amazement. The change to my body didn't happen overnight. It's been gradual, like the slow growth of hair over months and years. As I stare at my reflection in the mirror, it's difficult not to size myself up. I turn left and then right to see the shape of my protruding butt from both angles. The shorten mirror cuts my image in half, hiding the bottom. But my gaze is always in one place more than any other. I look down and fixate on my abdomen. For nearly fourteen years it has been the source of my pain and problems. It was often deflated, flattened from lack of food or nutrients. Friends used to surmise that I did sit-ups or stomach crunches; when in fact I rarely did either. My flat abdomen was primarily a result of my active colitis. When I met my partner three-and-a-half years ago, I remember he often commented on my flat stomach. When it was not flat, however, it was sick, bloated from gas or too much food from binging during short bouts of inactive disease, or the byproduct of menstruation. A bloated or full abdomen was previously not a healthy colon. In either form, flat or bloated, my colon was sick. But I knew it would always return to its flattened shape and my weight would remain under control by lost nutrients from loose stools and frequent bathroom visits. As I reminisce about my sick state, I briefly gaze into the mirror to see my abdomen in its present form: full, soft, and expansive as if flowing over my hips and extending down to my pelvis. I shake my head in disbelief and slight disgust as I turn my gaze toward the shower.

Temporal Comparison Theory (TCT) helps explain why this is a body I do not know, a body unrecognizable to myself. According to TCT, "people have a need to maintain a sense of self-continuity and self-consistency despite the fact that they are undergoing considerable change" (Klauer, Ferring and Filipp, 1998, p. 342). I did not acknowledge my body was experiencing anything other than a sick state for quite some time. I was primarily focused on my health and how I felt on the inside. It has only been more recently that I have begun to critically examine how I look, "the need to predict what lies ahead…" Klauer, Ferring and Filipp, 1998, p. 343), and cope with the loss of my sick self.

After a final rinse, I turn off the shower and reach outside the curtain for my blue towel, and start to dry off. I pass by the long hallway of mirrors in the bedroom and then by the closet doors and open the top dresser drawer. I grab a pair of underwear and slide them on, feeling the bottom half of my butt exposed because they no longer fit. I open the second drawer and reach for my shorts and slide one leg in after the other and up over my hips. As I zip the zipper, I notice the tightness around my abdomen as I pull the two sides together to button them. I sigh. This experience has become a regular part of my daily ritual; pants that barely fit. Last week I wore dress pants that were too tight for eight excruciatingly long hours, just to prove to myself I could still fit into them. With the bottom half of my body covered, I feel myself exhale and take a moment to pause and stare into the mirror above my dresser. I smile at my perky, forty-year-old breasts and defined shoulders and think, "Why on earth do we have so many mirrors in this place!?"

Part 2: Mirrored Reflections—Self Discrepancy Theory and Mirror Exposure

"Ouch. That hurt. No, I'm just kidding" he jokes, looking down as I gently pinch the skin around his waist. "What are you doing?" he asks kindly, yet inquisitively. "Look at this! See this here? When I pinch my skin I have a lot more than you do," I lament, letting go of my skin in disgust. "Women are supposed to have more curves than guys and more fat around their middle," my partner adds. "So you're calling me fat?" I laugh jokingly. "Of course not! I like your curves. It is part of being a woman," he smiles, pulling me closer. Medically, I know he's right. I know biologically women have higher concentrations of fat than men around their middle for childbearing. I know that the fat I carry is normal for a woman my size, shape, and age. I also know that I don't like it. It's not me. It's not who I am or who I was.

He runs his hands ever-so lightly across my belly and I flinch. I notice my immediate reaction to a simple, loving gesture. He is admiring me, loving me, and all I can do is think about my belly. I feel self-conscious in this moment because there is attention on my abdomen, the place where I observed and monitored its shape and internal movement for the past fourteen years. My colon lies deep inside, and for years has dictated and controlled what happens to the rest of me. I rarely let people touch my abdomen for fear that it might hurt. At times acting more like a turtle, I hunched over when I was actively ill to protect my soft underbelly from further harm. The conscious act of allowing someone to touch my abdomen is a gesture of trust, severe trust. In my current state, however, I am fearful of the ridicule for an out-of-control abdomen that seems to be taking on a shape of its own. As I move away again he asks, "What's wrong?" But he knows. He's touched my abdomen before and I've moved away. He knows I'm self-conscious. He knows I am embarrassed. My abdomen does not look like it once did. It does not act or behave as it once did. It does not feel like a part of me. I don't feel like myself. I have what psychologists refer to as self-discrepancy (Higgins, 1987). My actual/own self—as a present body in remission—is in contrast to my ideal/own self—my former ill body. Unlike the theory, as Higgins states, my ideal state is *not* in the future as something I hope to gain because I no longer wish to be sick. Rather, I wish to have the body I once knew simply because it is familiar and controllable to me. It is no wonder that I have such a strong emotional response to my actual-ideal discrepancy (Altabe and Thompson, 1996).

He kisses me gently and moves his hand down the front of my hip and I giggle, "You know I'm ticklish there." He smiles. As his hands continue to move across my back, shoulders, and legs, I glance in the mirror. There are three mirrors on both sides of our closets. Six opportunities to see my naked self. Having just gotten out of the shower and now standing in front of the mirrors, my body is on display, but I notice his eyes are tightly closed. My partner focuses his lips on my neck as he continues to move his hands down my back, and I continue to stare at the mirrored image of my body in front of me. I admire my long legs and the curve of my back. I consider what impact this mirror exposure might have on my body image disturbance (Delinsky and Wilson, 2006). I smile at our entwined bodies as we stand in this reflective embrace. We are rather beautiful together in our Greek statuesque pose, a slow-moving piece of art embodying admiration and love. But as he moves to draw his hands down my lower back, he reveals more of me, the middle section of my body is on display. My ribs, stomach, and abdomen are illuminated under the bright lights above. As if gazing at a grotesque image, I turn away and sigh. I kiss his neck and run my fingers across his shoulder blades trying to stay present, increasing the fervor of the moment. But my interest is waning because I am lost in my head. Lost in thoughts of self-ridicule and internalized critique. Lost in a state where I don't want to be, but cannot find my way out. The moment begins to slip away as I try desperately to stay focused, to stay in-the-moment. But I cannot stop as I lament about the thin, controlled body I once had.

Gazing Upon Venus: Flirting with Acceptance

The poster arrives in a prism-shaped cardboard cylinder, protecting the image inside. I am excited to open the tube and extract Venus from her encasing, but I have to go to the bathroom…again. Perhaps it's ironic or merely coincidental that since I began writing this chapter my colitis has flared in the past two days. I could write about my active colitis, but I've already done that in the past (Defenbaugh, 2008; Defenbaugh, 2013). This is the present. This is my "Colitis in Remission—with Bouts of Intermission" where I pause to run to a familiar place, the toilet. I have written so many things while sitting here including a majority of my book and previous articles, as well as the copious number of emails and Facebook posts. But today belongs to Venus.

I pick at the clear tape holding the two sides of the tube and begin ripping it across the fold. I finally open its shell and unfold the poster as the picture begins to emerge and she reveals herself to the light. I find myself fixated on Titian's *Venus of Urbino* (figure 2.2) and one feature in particular. She lays sprawled against a white sheet, unashamed about exposing her vulnerabilities, and aware she is being painted as a culturally beautiful woman from the fourteenth century. I briefly glance at the woman and young child in the background and notice the dog curled up near the foot of the bed. Nothing else catches my eye like the focus of her full abdomen. Like a fish hooked by a wire, my eyes are drawn to her midsection, the curvaceous shape of her abdomen, the section above where her hand rests (figure 2.3). I immediately wonder if she's pregnant, but the title of the piece reveals my error. The painter is attempting to capture the beauty of a young virgin who entices the viewer to gaze at her unabashed nakedness with desire and lust. She is an object to be admired and her features are to be revered. As the title also notes, the model is to be venerated for her beauty like the goddess Venus. The artist's emphasis of her youthful face and curvaceous figure highlight fourteenth century Italian cultural beliefs about women's bodies. In the painting we see weight equated with wealth and fertility, and beauty measured by the voluptuousness of a woman's sexual features.

I gaze again, a second, and then a third time, shaking my head at this illogical portrait of beauty. I recognize her youthfulness and nakedness were/are admired and that she embodies both financial wealth and aesthetic richness. She is the portrait of a goddess with an abdomen that is, quite frankly, unexplainable. My twenty-first century mind, brainwashed by excessive thinness and muscular physiques cannot fathom why her abdomen would be considered beautiful. Her remaining features are quite captivating, and I understand why Titian drew such a sensual and erotic picture. The portrait is alluring and overtly sexual even in this century, but it is her nakedness and not her specific features that I assume grab the attention of most viewers.

I cut the edges of the poster and frame her picture beneath cheap glass and a black plastic frame purchased at Wal-Mart. I place her picture in the window sill in my home office next to my desk. I want to understand why she is considered beautiful. I want to reframe my own thinking about beauty so that I can create a new identity and a more accepting belief about my body image. I gaze at Venus like one gazes at a thin portrayal of beauty in a TV ad. I can only hope that if I gaze at her image long enough, I will come to internalize this gaze and see myself as beautiful because I am healthy. Although I do not aspire to be viewed as an object of desire in the way the *Venus of Urbino* is portrayed, I do hope, one day, to look in the mirror and gaze upon myself with similar acceptance as a result of a shift in my self-perception.

Future: Uncertainty—A (Re)mission of Acceptance

In an Uncertain State of Remission: Remembering the Past to Face the Future

I have been in complete remission—minus an occasional short-term flare—for a number of years. You would think I know the exact number of years, months or even days; but I don't. I remember my last serious flare back in 2010 as a reaction to the antibiotics I took for my gum resection surgery which led to a two-month course of Azathioprine (immunosuppressant drug therapy). I remember other minor flares were due to bad food choices or were simply brought on by illness. My remission never lasted long and after nearly fourteen years after being diagnosed, you learn that having a chronic illness is just that, ongoing. You never settle in to the idea of remission. Unlike a warm blanket on a cold, winter evening, remission is more like a cool glass of water during a race. It offers temporary relief, but it never lasts long because you never stop running. Living with IBD is a lot like a marathon. You race to the bathroom, the doctor's office, and back to the bathroom. You race to pick up your medications and have your blood drawn for more tests. The chronicity of IBD is never ending and the moments of relief are often temporary.

I remember the first time I met someone in remission. I had been recently diagnosed with UC and decided to drive across the state, a couple of hours away to a Crohn's and Colitis Support group. I did not know anyone who was diagnosed with UC. I was lonely, afraid, and confused by this illness and fueled with a desire to learn more: an opportunity for my own personal knowledge and growth as well as fulfilling the requirements for my Ethnography graduate course. I drove to the community center and walked in where unfamiliar faces greeted me. Member after member slowly and painfully recounted their experiences. Their cases were often severe: bowel resections, colectomies, colostomies, ileostomies, and other IBD procedures. Most of the people in the group were diagnosed with Crohn's disease. It has been more than eleven years and although I don't remember all that was shared, I do remember one particular member of the group. She was an older woman in her late fifties or sixties. I remember her graying hair and flowing outfit. She embodied fluidity, softness, and groundedness. I also remember being frightened by the other members' stories, but when she spoke, she confidently and almost triumphantly announced "I've been in remission for a few decades now. Her words dropped like a bomb in a room filled with shattered memories or perhaps they were a ray of sunlight in a cavern of despair. She was the embodiment of possibility. I cannot recall her name or anything else she said, but I vividly remember her and the day I learned remission could be a reality.

I am now in a state of re-examining my internal locus of control (du Pré, 2014). In an ironic twist, I feel more out of control by the absence of managing and measuring my body. How bizarre. How truly bizarre. This is a new phase, a new body, a new life, a new perspective, a new salvaged identity (Charmaz, 1987) that is *not* a typical stage for a chronically ill existence. Remission is a prospect, a possibility that may happen but is unexpected and uncertain. According to Uncertainty Management Theory (Rains and Tukachinsky, 2015), I have a low level of desired uncertainty as a result of living with an unpredictable illness for more than a decade. Though I have come to find health uncertainty my "new norm," I still shy away from the unpredictability and favor the opportunities to control my illness and thus, control my health. I know very few people with IBD in long-term remission. And so I am left in what feels like a liminal space (Defenbaugh, 2011) of neither health nor illness. I feel healthy, but illness looms like a thunderstorm in the distance. Not knowing if it will pass, dissipate, bring rain, hail, damaging winds, or even death. There is too much uncertainty and this healthy state feels abnormal after so many years of chaos. The only thing I have known for the past fourteen years is that my state of health is not static. Change and uncertainty are certain. It will take time to establish a new normal, a new healthy state of mind and well-being.

CONCLUSION

Without an Ending: Returning to the Beginning

As a health communication scholar and feminist, I intended to write about what it means to embrace and accept a healthier body. But being in remission also means a shift in self-perception, a redefinition of normalcy, reflections of one's past, comparisons with the present and uncertainty about the future. Like others, chronic illness is "…marked by various critical events, remission or partial recovery periods, and comorbidities" (Donovan, Brown, LeFebvre, Tardif, Love, 2015, p. 703). This is a story about finding love for a body that feels out-of-control because my chronically ill parts are no longer weighed, measured, and regimented by high doses of steroids or anti-inflammatory medications. My body is no longer examined, poked, or prodded in the same way by members of the medical community. I now closely examine myself. I weigh and measure that which has become abnormal to my normal state of disease. The dis-ease I first felt having a chronic illness has become, after fourteen years, the norm of my identity and existence. Uncertainty is constant and stability is uncommon. I have come to identify myself as a chronically changing person. And so in this current state of remission, I do not know who I am, at least not yet. I only know who I was. I am shifting, once again, from one identity to another.

In the spirit of autoethnography and in writing about illness, I return to the beginning, choosing "resistance to finality and closure…" (Anderson and Glass-Coffin, 2013, p. 78). Choosing this story to exist in the "chronically liminal" space like Carol Rambo (2013) who struggles to find an ending and chooses to leave her story unresolved (p. 628). I too leave the story unresolved, waiting for the next healthy/ill/remission experience. I return to the beginning of this love story or rather, story about learning to love the (ill) self. The self that is still seen as ill and labeled as ill, but which continues to question, obscure, defy, and challenge standards of illness normativity by being in a chronic state of remission for an unknown period of time. And so…

> …I end the chapter where I began. I end returning to the self, returning to the . . . complex person I have become. I choose to end at the beginning of my continued quest. The journey is not over; it never is. It has only begun, once again. (Defenbaugh, 2011, p. 149)

REFERENCES

Altabe, M., and Thompson, J. K. (1996). "Body image: A cognitive self-schema construct?" *Cognitive Therapy and Research*, *20*(2), 171–193.

Anderson, J., and Bresnahan, M. (2013). "Communicating stigma about body size." *Health Communication*, *28*(6), 603–615.

Anderson, L., and Glass-Coffin, B. (2013). "I learn by going: Autoethnographic modes of inquiry." In S. H. Jones, T.E. Adams, & C. Ellis (Eds.), *Handbook of autoethnography* (pp. 57–83). London: Routledge.

Chang, H. (2008). *Autoethnography as method.* Walnut Creek, CA: Left Coast Press.

Charmaz, K (1987). "Struggling for a self: Identity levels of the chronically ill." In J. Roth and P. Conrad (Eds.), *Research in the Sociology of Health Care* (pp. 282–321). Greenwich, CT: JAI Press.

Chen, Y., and Feeley, T. H. (2014). "Numeracy, information seeking, and self-efficacy in managing health: An analysis using the 2007 Health Information National Trends Survey (HINTS)." *Health Communication, 29*(9), 843–853.

da Silva, G. M., Hull, T., Roberts, P. L., Ruiz, D. E., Wexner, S. D., Weiss, E. G., et al. (2008). "The effect of colorectal surgery in female sexual function, body image, self-esteem and general health: A prospective study." *Annals of Surgery*, *248*(2), 266–272.

Davis, C., and Quinlan, M. Communicating stigma and acceptance. In J. Yamasaki, P. Geist-Martin, and B. F. Sharf (Eds.), *Storied health and illness: Communicating personal, cultural, & political complexities* (pp. 191–220). Long Grove, IL: Waveland Press.

Defenbaugh, N. L. (2008). "'Under erasure': The absent ill body in doctor—patient dialogue." *Qualitative Inquiry,14*(8), 1402–1424.

Defenbaugh, N. L. (2011). *Dirty tale: A narrative journey of the IBD body*. New York: Hampton Press.

Defenbaugh. N. (2013). "Revealing and concealing ill identity: A performance narrative of IBD disclosure." *Health Communication, 28*(2), 159–169. DOI: 10.1080/10410236.2012.666712

Delinsky, S. S., & Wilson, G. T. (2006). "Mirror exposure for the treatment of body image disturbance." *International Journal of Eating Disorders*, *39*(2), 108–116.

De Rooy, E. C., Toner, B. B., Maunder, R. G., Greenberg, G. R., Baron, D., Steinhart, A. H., et al. (2001). "Concerns of patients with inflammatory bowel disease: Results from a clinical population." *The American Journal of Gastroenterology*, *96*(6), 1816–1821.

Donovan, E. E., Brown, L. E., LeFebvre, L., Tardif, S., and Love, B. (2015). "'The uncertainty is What is driving me crazy': The tripartite model of uncertainty in the adolescent and young adult cancer context." *Health Communication, 30*(7), 702–713.

Drossman, D. A., Patrick, D. L., Mitchell, C. M., Zagami, E. A., and Appelbaum, M. I. (1989). "Health related quality of life in inflammatory bowel disease." *Digestive Diseases and Sciences, 34*(9), 1379–1386.

du Pré, A. (2014)(4th ed.). *Communicating about health: Current issues and perspectives.* Oxford University Press.

Gallagher, S. (1986). "Body image and body schema: A conceptual clarification." *Journal of Mind and Behavior, 7*(4), 541–554.

Goffman, E. (1963). "Stigma: Notes on the management of spoiled identity." Englewood: Prentice Hall.

Gutzmer, K., and Beach, W. A. (2015). "'Having an ovary this big is not normal': Physicians' use of normal to assess wellness and sickness during oncology interviews." *Health Communication, 30*(1), 8–18.

Higgins, E. T. (1987). "Self-discrepancy: A theory relating self and affect." *Psychological Review, 94*(3), 319.

Howes, H. F. R., Edwards, S., and Benton, D. (2005). "Female body image following acquired brain injury." *Brain Injury, 19*(6), 403–415.

Klauer, T., Ferring, D., and Filipp, S. H. (1998). "'Still stable after all this...?': Temporal comparison in coping with severe and chronic disease." *International Journal of Behavioral Development, 22*(2), 339–355.

Knowles, S. R., Gass, C., and Macrae, F. (2013). "Illness perceptions in IBD influence psychological status, sexual health and satisfaction, body image and relational functioning: A preliminary exploration using structural equation modeling." *Journal of Crohn's and Colitis, 7*(9), e344-e350.

Larson, D. W., Davies, M. M., Dozois, E. J., Cima, R. R., Piotrowicz, K., Anderson, K., et al. (2008). "Sexual function, body image, and quality of life after laparoscopic and open ileal pouch-anal anastomosis. *Diseases of the Colon and Rectum, 51*(4), 392–396.

Lockford, L. (2014). "Trusting the bridging power of autoethnography." *International Review of Qualitative Research,7*(3), 283–289.

Muller, K. R., Prosser, R., Bampton, P., Mountifield, R., and Andrews, J. M. (2010). "Female gender and surgery impair relationships, body image, and sexuality in inflammatory bowel disease: Patient perceptions." *Inflammatory Bowel Diseases, 16*(4), 657–663.

Rains, S. A., and Tukachinsky, R. (2015). "An examination of the relationships among uncertainty, appraisal, and information-seeking behavior proposed in uncertainty management theory." *Health Communication, 30*(4), 339–349.

Rambo, C. (2013). "Twitch: A Performance of Chronic Liminality." In Jones, S. H., Adams, T. E., & Ellis, C. (Eds.), *Handbook of Autoethnography* (pp. 627–638). London: Routledge.

Richards, R. (2008). "Writing the othered self: Autoethnography and the problem of objectification in writing about illness and disability." *Qualitative Health Research, 18*(12), 1717–1728.

Thompson, J. K., and Stice, E. (2001). "Thin-ideal internalization: Mounting evidence for a new risk factor for body-image disturbance and eating pathology." *Current Directions in Psychological Science, 10*(5), 181–183.

UCSF Medical Center (2016). "Special concerns for people with j-pouches." Retrieved on September 29, 2016 fromhttps://www.ucsfhealth.org/education/special_concerns_for_people_with_j-pouches/.

White, C. A. (2000). "Body image dimensions and cancer: A heuristic cognitive behavioral model." *Psycho-Oncology, 9*(3), 183–192.

Wikipedia (2005). "Remission in Medicine." Retrieved on September 30, 2016 fromhttp://www.dictionary.com/browse/remission?s=t.

Yamasaki, J., Geist-Martin, P., and Sharf, B. F. (2017). *Storied health and illness: Communicating personal, cultural, and political complexities.* Long Grove, IL: Waveland Press.

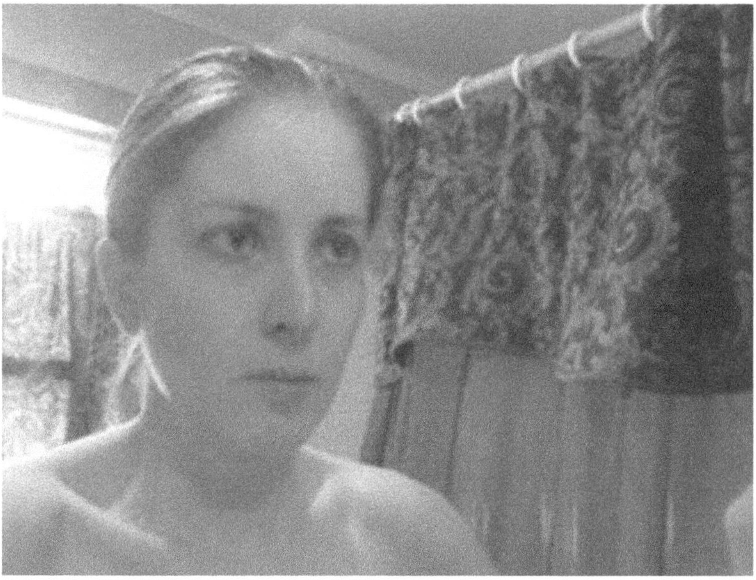

Figure 2.1. Performance Art—"The Reality: Memoir of a Colon." Photo taken by the author (2011) and uploaded to Facebook.

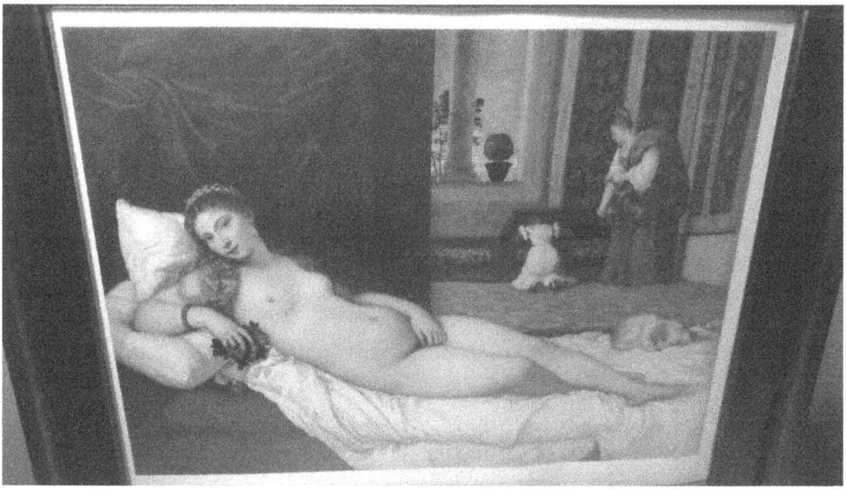

Figure 2.2. *Venus of Urbino* by Titian, 1538. Photo taken by the author.

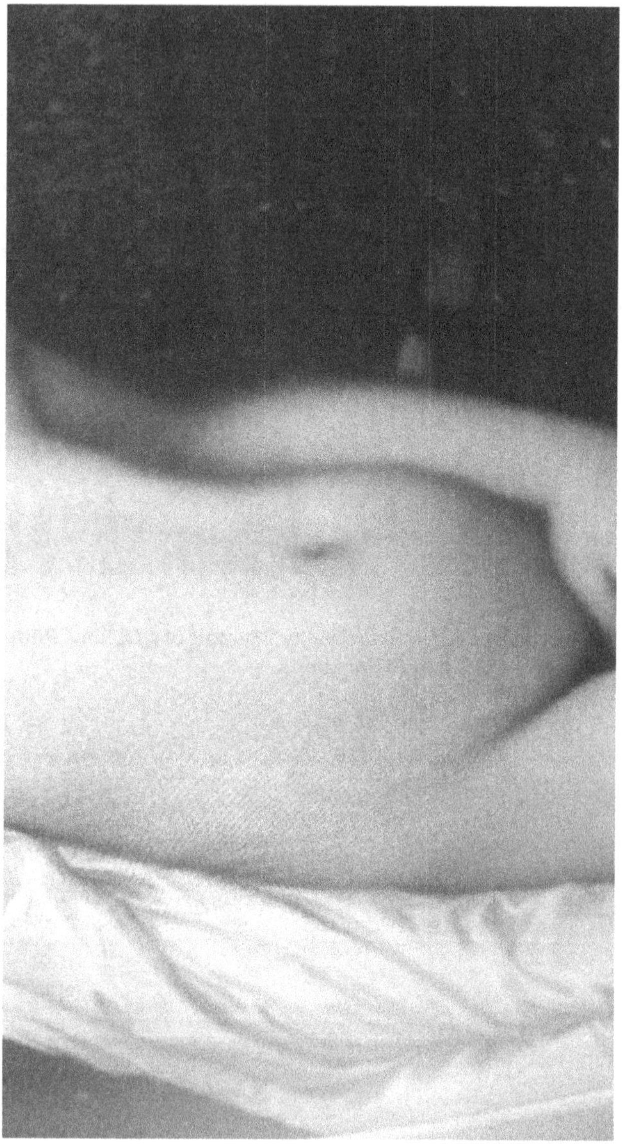

Figure 2.3. Detail of *Venus of Urbino* by Titian, 1538. Photo taken by the author.

Chapter Three

A Semblance of Normalcy

Social Isolation and the Burden of Looking Well

Hannah Thyberg

It was November, and I was curled up on the cold, unfriendly tile of the bathroom. The fluorescent light glared unforgivingly, furrowing its eyebrows in disgust. The mold-stained shower curtain was partially pulled back, revealing a pathetic drip from the faucet head and a clump of my suitemate's dark, matted hair, sprouting from the drain like weeds. Tears streamed down my cheeks. Even my fingernails ached. My soul quivered like an overstrained muscle. I couldn't hold on anymore.

This wasn't the first time I had found myself sitting on the shower floor, and it certainly wouldn't be the last. Yet it was a definitive moment for me nonetheless because at that moment I knew in the deepest part of me that something was undeniably wrong, that I had finally reached my breaking point. I ended my first semester of college in a daze, numb to the life around me. And then I went home, where I spent the following semester lying on the couch instead of at school. And so began my journey with chronic illness.

Let's rewind a few months. I was a recent high school graduate about to start my freshman year in college. I went off to school with apprehension and anticipation, about to embark on the most exciting and formative years of my life. I had been told time and again that college was a place of self-discovery, a time to explore the world, make friends, and broaden your horizons. I set out with high, albeit uncertain, expectations for the next four years, never guessing what my journey would entail.

It was subtle at first, little things, things that could easily be brushed off or explained away; the occasional ache or twinge. My joints felt stiff. Then came the headaches. I started to feel more tired from day to day. Everything seemed to require a lot of effort. Individually, my symptoms seemed relatively benign, easily attributable to regular things like stress or studying, or perhaps sitting too long in class. I chalked it up to the "growing pains" of college, which after all was a major life transition.

And then it became less subtle. What started out as occasional and brief became more intense and more frequent. My energy continued to plummet. I wasn't able to make it up a flight of stairs without getting winded and needing a break. I couldn't even make it through a shower without having to sit down. I felt poorly for larger and larger portions of the day. Eventually, I'd wake up feeling ill, and that sick feeling would last the entire day. I began to have more bad days than good days, days when it took everything I had just to stumble out of bed and make it to class. Then came the days where I couldn't make it out of bed at all. As my lethargy mounted, I fell further and further behind. To this day I still don't know how I survived, let alone passed my first semester. At the end of four excruciating months, I packed my belongings up and returned to Pittsburgh, utterly defeated.

The first few weeks were spent in a stuporous state of hibernation. I became intimately familiar with the texture and pattern of my sofa cushions. Too tired to even watch TV, I simply vegetated in a pathetic state of malaise. After a brief catatonic stint, I began to seek medical help. The diagnostic process was grueling. I spent countless hours in doctor's offices, being poked and prodded and asked over and over again to explain, "what was wrong with me." I was shuffled between specialists, lab techs, and phlebotomists, all of whom came to the same unsatisfactory conclusion. I'd get a skeptical look from over the top of a clipboard and hear those five gut-wrenching words: "We can't find anything wrong." Some were more apologetic than others; some were less than subtle about their conviction that it was all in my head. But all were unable to offer any explanation as to why I felt this way.

I slid into a place of bitter dejection. My situation felt completely hopeless, and I could see no light at the end of the tunnel. I was trapped. Peterson (2012) aptly describes this feeling of disconsolation, writing:

> When you're weak, it can feel as if you have no choices—as if all doors are closed, all windows are shut, all avenues of escape have been blocked. You have no choice in anything. Instead, things just happen to you. This, by the way, is a lie. While the range of your choices may be limited when you are weak, this does not mean that you have no choices at all. It's just that your choices might be difficult to see, and may, indeed, seem too small or too inconsequential to be of value. (p. 8)

At the time I was unable to see my choices. I had no tangible sense of agency. Instead, I was entirely focused on my feelings of victimization. All I saw was my lack of control. All I felt was disempowered. I was completely at the mercy of modern medicine, and that medicine was failing me.

After what seemed like an unending series of appointments, I was finally referred to a rheumatologist. I remember sitting in his office feeling that same tiredness, the heavy weight of anticipated disappointment. Why would this appointment be any different than the other dead ends before it? The doctor entered the room, greeted me, and proceeded to ask the standard questions. After conversing for a few minutes, he completed a physical exam, as well as something known as a Tender Point Survey. "This survey is a notation of pain response to careful palpation of specific body locations using a light compression" (Jones and Hoffman, 2009, p. 7). It involves a total of eighteen tender-point locations, with reported tenderness in at least eleven of eighteen points being considered a positive test (Barker, 2005). It was very brief, uneventful even—I tested positive for all eighteen spots. When the doctor turned to face me, I felt that familiar sinking feeling in my gut, the one that told me there must not be anything wrong if he'd already given up. But to my surprise, what came out of his mouth was something completely different than I had heard before. He explained that his findings were consistent with something called fibromyalgia.

Most individuals with chronic illness will agree that there is some form of relief when an actual diagnosis is found. Having an official name not only helps a person to organize her complaints and more intelligibly explain her suffering, but it also "holds the promise of reincorporating the sufferer into the social world from which she has been alienated" (Barker, 2005, p. 112). Naming a disease or illness confirms that there was, in fact, something wrong and that the person isn't just crazy. A positive diagnosis confirms rather than contradicts the individual's subjective experience. As Barker (2005) writes:

> A diagnosis represents the physician's comprehension of the patient's experience. Importantly, a diagnosis gives the physician a medical plan of action to treat or aid the patient in his or her return to health. For the patient, a diagnosis gives meaning and legitimacy to worrying symptoms and provides a framework for what he or she is facing. For all these reasons, when a patient presents distressing symptoms to a physician, both parties may find even a bad diagnosis to be better than no diagnosis at all. (p. 20)

I remember that feeling of relief as if my entire body let out a collective sigh of palliation. After all this time I finally had an answer, a tangible name to assign to my affliction. And yet, with this answer came a whole slew of new, unanswered questions. What was fibromyalgia? Was it treatable? Was I dying? How did it start? My mind quickly transitioned from relief to racing panic. I didn't know how to slow my thoughts down enough to respond coherently to the doctor's pronouncement. Thankfully, he wasn't fazed by my shocked silence and took it upon himself to provide a general overview. And so, in the span of a half hour, I went from being a hypochondriacal teenager to someone with a confirmed, legitimate illness.

The name fibromyalgia comes from the medical root words: *fibra* (fiber), *myo* (muscle), and *algos* (pain) (Jones and Hoffman, 2009). As Barker (2005) explains, fibromyalgia is not so much a disease as a syndrome of symptoms, "such as chronic, widespread pain...fatigue, headaches, sleep irregularities, irritable bowel syndrome, irritable bladder syndrome, cognitive and mood disorders, and increased sensitivity to stimuli" (p. 3). It is most commonly characterized by unexplained, chronic, widespread pain (Ostalecki, 2008). This diffuse musculoskeletal pain is often accompanied by persistent fatigue and generalized stiffness (Barker, 2005). Another hallmark symptom of fibromyalgia is something they call "fibro fog." As Jones and Hoffman (2009) explain, this can include difficulty thinking or multi-tasking, as well as difficulty with cognition and short-term recall. Other memory related problems associated with fibro fog include difficulty paying attention, forgetfulness, disorientation when driving, and difficulty remembering names and faces (Ali, 2016).

Fibromyalgia is still not fully understood. However, the heightened experience of pain is believed to come from "an amplification of pain processing and defects in pain inhibition in the central nervous system—a phenomenon called 'central sensitization'" (Berne, 2002, p. 26). This hypersensitization leads to *allodynia*—the sensation of pain felt in the absence of a painful stimulus, and *hyperalgesia*—a heightened pain response to a stimulus that normally causes only minor pain (Berne, 2002). In addition to heightening the experience of painful stimuli, central sensitization causes amplification of other sensory stimuli. Ostalecki (2008) likens this to having the volume knob of your sensory world perpetually turned up. Temperatures, sounds, smells, and light are all magnified.

All medical jargon aside, it basically boiled down to feeling tired and achy almost all the time. Everything hurt and my whole body felt heavy as if my skin was made of the same stuff as the thick lead vests they make you wear at the dentist's office whenever you get an x-ray. It felt like having the flu round the clock. As the rheumatologist explained, I had it "in spades," meaning I was a regular poster child for fibromyalgia.

I had all the classic signs and symptoms, including being female. According to Jones and Hoffman (2009), women are eight to nine times more likely than men to be diagnosed with fibromyalgia. Some estimates suggest that as many as ninety percent of diagnosed cases are female (Sheehan, 2012). It is still unclear as to why women are more commonly afflicted than men. Current thinking suggests it is a combination of biology, psychology, and sociocultural factors. A common theory focuses on the production of hormones. Women produce much higher levels of estrogen than men. Furthermore, these levels fluctuate throughout the month. Many women report cyclical worsening of symptoms that align with the dips in estrogen production caused by menstruation. (Sheehan, 2012). Estrogen is believed to be protective against pain. Thus lower levels would presumably be associated with worsening pain symptoms. Additionally, men are believed to more effectively produce endorphins, "natural substances in the brain that activate its pain-killing receptors" (Sheehan, 2012). This increases their overall pain threshold in comparison to women.

In regards to non-biological theories, researchers suggest that the social perception of pain between genders may influence the prevalence of pain disorders. The experience of pain is considered more socially acceptable among females, whereas males are more commonly expected to exhibit toughness and stoicism (Matallana, 2017). As a result, male sufferers may hide or deny pain in an effort to maintain a socially appropriate gender role. Other thinking suggests that because fibromyalgia has come to be viewed as a primarily "female problem," male patients may be overlooked. In other words, medical providers may be less likely to consider it as a possible diagnosis. Still, others suggest that males may seek medical advice less frequently, and thus are less likely to be diagnosed in the first place (Sheehan, 2012).

Though my gender was typical, my age was not. Despite having all the classic symptoms, I am considered an unusual case, as I developed the condition substantially earlier than the average patient. Fibromyalgia is most commonly diagnosed in middle age (Jones and Hoffman, 2009). To be diagnosed right after high school was very rare. Truth be told, this incredibly disheartened me. It made me feel like a freak. Why was I so different? My only consolation was that despite fibromyalgia being a persistent, often lifelong condition, it was not considered degenerative or fatal (Berne, 2002).

My young age was one of the reasons it had been so difficult to find a diagnosis. Not only that, but as Ostalecki (2008) explains, fibromyalgia is somewhat slippery to diagnose, in that it can mirror or coexist with other conditions such as chronic fatigue syndrome, rheumatoid arthritis, hypothyroidism, irritable bowel syndrome, or depression. Furthermore, fibromyalgia lacks more concrete testing or screening processes and is often diagnosed based on more subjective experiences than quantitative measures. Hester (2015) writes:

> In the absence of definitive medical tests for some invisible illnesses, such as fibromyalgia, patients fight to be taken at their word—to have doctors, friends, and family believe that they're reliable narrators of their own experiences… The burden of proof often falls squarely on the ill person. (para. 8)

I certainly experienced this. Throughout the entire process, it felt as if I were on trial, desperately trying to convince my doctors that there was, in fact, something wrong with me. My symptoms were vague and scattered. They didn't align with a positive diagnosis according to any standard medical test. Until the rheumatologist, it appeared as if I was simply conjuring up maladies. It was a huge step forward to have a confirmed diagnosis. Yet my journey was far from over.

Following my diagnosis, I spent the next several months learning about fibromyalgia and what it means to live with this condition. I read books, met with more specialists, and even attended an outpatient pain clinic. I was the youngest group member at the clinic by several decades. I remember the dubious looks of suspicion and surprise, as people three times my age listened to my story. I was an anomaly: young but not healthy, sick but not old. I didn't fit in, even here—the place where people came to gain a sense of camaraderie from others with similar physical realities. I was the odd one out—in a completely different stage of life, with totally different needs and concerns. That freakish insecure feeling rose in me yet again. I started to feel like no one would ever be able to relate to me. After all, it seemed like I was the one and only person in the world who was like this.

I returned to school the next fall, eager to regain some semblance of "normalcy," yet I had tremendous anxiety about whether I'd be able to handle it. After all, my first college attempt hadn't gone too smoothly. Not only was I nervous about the more pragmatic, academic side of things, I was also uneasy about how I would fit in among my peers. I hadn't done a great job of making close friends in my first semester and certainly hadn't kept in touch with any classmates during my time off. Would they be glad to see me again? Would they even remember me? How would I explain where I had been the last semester? I felt awkward and defensive, uncertain of what or how much to say.

During my first week back I had a striking interaction with a classmate that I will never forget. I was walking across campus when I heard someone call my name. I turned around to see a former classmate. We quickly exchanged greetings, and then he said, rather emphatically, "You're wearing real pants! I almost didn't recognize you without your pajamas." Although the underlying intent of his comment was lighthearted, I remember feeling utterly crushed by his words. I was devastated to realize that I had earned the reputation of being "the pajama girl." I felt embarrassed and ridiculous for being unrecognizable in normal human adult attire. How pathetic was I that it was noteworthy for me to wake up and put on pants in the morning? I felt like I was back in kindergarten; here's a gold star for being a big girl! It was completely infantilizing.

Not all my interactions were as noteworthy. In fact, most of my conversations felt eerily similar, as if I had landed myself a role as Bill Murray in *Groundhog Day*. They all entailed some superficial attempt to casually explain my absence, some brief recitation about how I had been feeling sick, but things were "more under control now." And that was as far as I let it go.

It was draining, but somehow it seemed easier that way, so I did my best to keep a smile on my face whenever possible.

The fact that the sequencing of my courses was now a semester behind further complicated my transition back to school. My schedule was a strange hybrid of freshman and sophomore courses. As such, I didn't fit into a cohort anymore. A few of my classes were with my original freshman class. But the other half was with the cohort below me. This left me in an awkward position. I wasn't really a part of either group, just a weird drifter who floated between the two. The classmates I started out with had gone through an entire semester without me, one full of memories and deepened friendships, all of which I simply wasn't a part of. The new cohort had spent the entire week before the start of the semester on a camping trip, an experience intentionally designed to help students bond quickly. Again I found myself walking into a group of people with a unique set of shared experiences, inside jokes, and cliques, with no space to fit into. Again I was in a position where I didn't fully belong. It was incredibly lonely.

That feeling of loneliness overshadowed most of my college experience. Some things got easier with time, and I did eventually make some friends. But I also spent a substantial amount of time on my own. I wasn't on any sports teams or in any clubs. Most of my weekends were spent traveling back home for doctor's appointments. If I was in town, I usually skipped social functions because I was too tired or in too much pain. I didn't pull all-nighters studying with classmates because my body simply couldn't handle it. I lived in a singles dormitory. I even avoided the cafeteria because the noise and crowds were over-stimulating. As a result, I missed out on a lot of the traditional college experience. This only further substantiated the feeling that I was different. It seemed that a precedent had been set early on that I would never really fit in. I would always be, in some sense, a loner. So I got accustomed to living a somewhat isolated life. I recall a professor commenting on this one day. She remarked, "whenever I see you, you're just always doing your own thing." It seemed even the staff took note that I spent most of my time on my own; whether it was walking to and from class, or sitting alone in the library studying, it wasn't often that I had company.

Navigating the social dynamic with my peers was only half the battle. I was still faced with the challenge of surviving the academic portion of college. My physical health played a huge role in this. I had difficulty attending class at times when I was in too much pain. I remember times when I had to put my head down during class or lay down in the back of the classroom with my eyes closed because the fluorescent lights gave me headaches. I had to register through the student center for special needs accommodations. At the beginning of each semester, I gave my professors a medical excuse from my doctor explaining my condition. I met with each of them to explain why I would require extra absences, testing accommodations, or extensions on assignments at times. I felt incredibly awkward during these meetings. I wanted to keep my life private, and it was uncomfortable sharing such personal information with so many people. It was difficult to come to terms with the necessity of this transparency. I needed to advocate for myself in order to be successful, which required vulnerability. However, I couldn't shake that feeling of embarrassment for needing special treatment.

Though I found that most of the staff was willing to work with me, it was an arduous process that added another burden to my education. Not only did it require time and effort to complete the necessary paperwork, but it created yet another relational dynamic where I felt insecure and abnormal. I wasn't just another student—I was the student with the special needs. It seemed that every level of my college experience was affected by this feeling of separateness, with the compound total creating a pervasive pattern of isolation.

The introversion I developed in college has only continued in my years since graduation. I still spend a considerable amount of time by myself. I struggle to participate in social activities, not only because I feel socially awkward, but also because I have no idea on any given day how I'm going to feel or whether or not I'll be up for it. This makes it incredibly difficult to commit to anything in advance because I can't guarantee that I'll be able to follow through when the time finally comes. The reality is that I have limited control of my body. Whether it's due to extreme exhaustion or a blinding headache, there have been numerous occasions when I've had to cancel plans at the last minute because I simply don't have the physical capacity to participate. It's discouraging—not only the feeling of lack of control but the feeling that I am in some way a disappointment to others. I hate letting people down. I hate not keeping promises. Donoghue and Siegel (1992) summarize it well, writing:

> The planning that most of us do naturally, the patient of ICI [invisible chronic illness] does with an ominous sense of whistling in the dark. This inability to plan ahead severely limits personal enjoyment and achievement and greatly strains social life and relationships… This interpersonal strain is part of the difficulty in adjusting to the chronicity of the illness. (p. 59)

For a time I tried to commit to things anyway and simply force myself to power through. The results were abysmal. I was utterly miserable the entire time, which made me terrible company. I'd be painfully self-conscious, overcome by a powerful sense of insecurity, as I tried desperately to keep up appearances and hide just how badly I felt. I resented everyone in the room, including myself. As if that wasn't bad enough, there would always be an extended recovery period after the fact. It took days to regroup from the strain of forced socialization. As you can imagine, it simply wasn't sustainable.

So instead I've become one of those noncommittal people who is always vague and ambiguous about plans, saying "maybe" or "we'll see" or "I'll try." Although it has never been said outright, I'm convinced that people perceive me as a complete flake. I have friends who have just stopped inviting me to things altogether because they don't expect me to come. It's discouraging, especially because I largely feel misunderstood.

I suppose you're asking yourself why I don't just explain myself to others. But the truth is, I never really talk about my illness because I don't know how. Frankly, it feels futile even to try. Defenbaugh (2013) comments that it is often easier to conceal illness than it is to exert the time and effort it takes to reveal. As a sufferer of ulcerative colitis, Defenbaugh (2013) herself is an expert in the "art of concealment," and discusses the great lengths she has gone to in order to maintain "a healthy look at all costs" (p. 164). There are limited arenas where it feels safe or appropriate to disclose the details of one's illness. Thus, sufferers compensate for the difficulty of being "flung [into] the land of healthy normalcy" by restricting or minimizing what they disclose (Defenbaugh, 2013, p. 165). For example, I can share the more clinical aspects with my family and my doctors, but I can never delve past the superficial nature of my experience. Frank (1991) captures this beautifully, writing:

> We have plenty of words to describe specific pains: sharp, throbbing, piercing, burning, even dull. But these words do not describe the experience of pain. We lack terms to express what it means to live "in" such pain. Unable to express pain, we come to believe there is nothing to say. Silenced, we become isolated in pain, and the isolation increases the pain. Like the sick feeling that comes with the recognition of yourself as ill, there is a pain attached to being in pain. (p. 29–30)

Talking about invisible illness is challenging because "symptoms of invisible chronic illnesses are not only non-observable, but also typically immeasurable. They are subjective experiences" (Donoghue and Siegel, 1992, p. 7). People living with invisible illness don't adhere to an easily recognizable schema. There is a pronounced disconnect between the internally lived experience and the externally perceived reality. On the outside, everything appears to be fine, healthy, normal. But underneath the façade of normalcy is an entirely different reality. The sick person looks "well" but, in fact, is not. These false appearances hurt the ability of both the individuals and others to trust that an actual problem exists. As a result, people with invisible illness are frequently under suspicion from others, and sometimes even themselves, that the condition is psychological (Donoghue and Siegel, 1992). Thus, "relationships and social interactions are constantly burdened by the sufferers' appearance of well-being" (Barker, 2005, p. 127).

Donoghue and Siegel (1992) pose that “the human potential to reach out in care seems to be tapped particularly when the need for the other is indisputably apparent” (p. 3). They continue to explain that “the symptoms of invisible illness have no external evidence of suffering that elicits compassion. Instead, the patient often endures suspicion and withdrawal from others” (Donoghue and Siegel, 1992, p. 4–5). In other words, people aren’t naturally inclined to offer sympathy or compassion to those with an invisible illness. Rather, they are more likely to seek proof or justification to substantiate your claim of being ill. This is perhaps the most hurtful aspect of living with invisible illness. It’s frustrating to feel as if you have to justify yourself to others. The burden of proof is just another weight to an already heavy experience.

To add insult to injury, people often forget that you’re ill, even if you’ve told them before. It’s happened to me more times than I can count—with people who I’ve known for years, people I’ve dated, even my own family. On some level I understand it’s not their fault; after all, it isn’t readily apparent, nor does it impact them personally. So it’s only natural that they wouldn’t remember. But I find myself feeling bitter, nonetheless, that they have the privilege to forget. Individuals with chronic illness “cannot move or breathe or have a life without our illness showing its control over our body. It puts us in the position of fighting for everything” (Copen, 2015). There isn’t a day or moment of my life that I get to escape from that reality. Each reminder to them serves as a painful reminder to myself. I hear that small voice in my head say, “You’re sick. You’re different. No one understands you. You’ll never belong.”

In writing this chapter, one of the critical elements I’ve had to consider is just how exactly I hold my illness. From the start, I knew that social isolation was a predominant theme in my life and that it would have some part in my narrative. But as I began to flesh out the idea of isolation, I realized it was somewhat superficial. There was a deeper undercurrent beneath my feelings of loneliness and isolation, and it stemmed from the core foundation of how I view myself and what it means to be ill. If I am brutally honest, my personal understanding of illness is an incredibly negative one. It’s hard for me to admit, but in some sense, I think I look down on my illness. My most fundamental understanding of illness is that it is a flaw, a defect, an imperfection—something that must be apologized and compensated for. Although this understanding is largely subconscious, it has greatly influenced how I live my life. It’s why I try so hard to keep up social appearances, to deny, in some way, that I’m sick.

The cold, hard truth is that I am ashamed of my body. I am embarrassed to share with others that I struggle with a chronic condition. I’m afraid of being looked down on. I’m afraid of people thinking that I’m somehow less than everybody else. I’m afraid of being reduced to my illness, confined and constrained by one aspect of my life rather than who I am as a whole. Because when you're sick, sometimes it feels like that's all you are. You're no longer a woman, or a writer, or a sister, or a chocolate enthusiast. You're just sick.

To protect and maintain my pride, I've invested a tremendous amount of time and energy trying to combat that "sickly" image. Not just for the sake of others, but for mine as well. There are still days when I'm in complete denial, because more than anything, I hate the feeling of limitation. Although I've been living with fibromyalgia for several years now, there are still days when I struggle to accept my normal. I am still angry, bitter, tearful, and exasperated. There are still times when all I can see is what I don't have, what I don't get to do or be. I still feel the stinging loss of how things should have been. And I mourn.

Time has taught me that there are some things you never get over, but that you just have to get through. There's no magical switch or transition where you suddenly become happy, let alone cured. It's not a linear path. It's a chaotic cycle that varies with each season of life. In the words of Frank (1991):

> Doing with the body is only part of what needs to be done for the person. What happens when my body breaks down happens not just to that body but also to my life, which is lived in that body. When the body breaks down, so does the life. Even when medicine can fix the body, that doesn't always put the life back together again. Medicine can diagnose and treat the breakdown, but sometimes so much fear and frustration have been aroused in the ill person that fixing the breakdown does not quiet them. At those times the experience of illness goes beyond the limits of medicine. (p. 8)

Perhaps this is why I became a nurse; to offer more than mere medicine. I understand the chaos and complexity of what it is to be ill, to hurt, what it is to be at the mercy of someone's care and understanding. I have ached for consolation and comfort on countless occasions, never knowing how to ask for it. Though I struggle to this day to seek it out, what I have found in myself is a capacity to offer unto others what I have yearned for, to extend compassion in times of need and vulnerability. I love what I do. It is a privilege to meet people where they are and to acknowledge the fullest, truest versions of who they are. And in so doing, I am learning each day how to better meet myself.

REFERENCES

Ali, N. (2016). *Understanding fibromyalgia*. Lanham, MD: Rowan & Littlefield.

Barker, K. K. (2005). *The fibromyalgia story: Medical authority and women's worlds of pain*. Philadelphia, PA: Temple University Press.

Berne, K. (2002). *Chronic fatigue syndrome, fibromyalgia and other invisible illnesses: The comprehensive guide*. Alameda, CA: Hunter House Inc.

Copen, L. (2015, September 23). "Invisible illness or chronic illness? What's the difference?" *The Huffington Post.* Retrieved from http://www.huffingtonpost.com/lisa-copen/invisible-illness_b_8178886.html

Defenbaugh, N. L. (2013). "Revealing and concealing ill identity: A performance narrative of IBD disclosure." *Health Communication, 28*, 159–169. DOI: 10.1080/10410236.2012.666712

Donoghue, P. J., and Siegel, M. E. (1992). *Sick and tired of feeling sick and tired.* New York, NY: W.W. Norton & Company.

Frank, A.W. (1991). *At the will of the body: Reflections on illness.* Boston, MA: Houghton Mifflin Company.

Hester, J. L. (2015). "Living with invisible illness." *The Atlantic.* Retrieved from http://www.theatlantic.com/health/archive/2015/07/invisible-illness-chronic-disease-fibromyalgia/398393/

Jones, K. D., and Hoffman, J. H. (2009). *Fibromyalgia.* Santa Barbara, CA: Greenwood Press.

Matallana, L. (2017). *Women and pain: A focus on fibromyalgia.* Retrieved from http://www.fmaware.org/about-fibromyalgia/prevalence/women-fibro/

Ostalecki, S. (2008). *Fibromyalgia: The complete guide from medical experts and patients.* Sudbury, MA: Jones and Bartlett Publishers.

Peterson, D. N. (2012). "Choosing weakness." *The Covenant Companion*, February, 6–9.

Sheehan, J. (2012). "The role of gender in fibromyalgia." Retrieved from http://www.everydayhealth.com/fibromyalgia/101/the-role-of-gender.aspx

Chapter Four

Transparency and Disclosure

Tools for Building Trust and Confidence

Emily Pfender

The prick of a needle wakes me each morning. Vitals. Pills. Pressure to conform. I want to resist. I want to fight. I want to scream, but I want to go home more. Perplexed physicians express confusion over my admission; to them, I appear stable. So why do I feel like a guinea pig in the throes of a science experiment? My hair, unkempt and knotted, smells like *old lady shampoo.* No personal hairbrush, deodorant, or shampoo because the medical team is concerned I might swallow them in an effort to kill myself. I try to convince them that I will not hurt myself *here*, but they will not take my words as truth. After all, I am in a psychiatric hospital.

I closely watch the hands of the clock; time passing slowly. It is almost visiting hour, and my dad and brother are coming to see me this evening. The designated visitor room looks like a middle school lunchroom, filled with round tables and chairs. I slump lower into my chair, rewrapping myself in the blanket from my assigned room as my dad and brother enter. They are searched and patted down by staff and are required to turn in all personal items—cell phones, wallets, and anything else they were carrying. They enter the room and walk toward me. As they approach, I remain sitting, bundled up in my blanket. My brother's warm smile greets me as they approach. I smile back. "You don't belong here, Emily," says my father. Thinking back to that moment, I cannot remember how I responded to his comment, but most likely it was with irritation because I often receive this reaction from those around me. Family, psychologists, psychiatrists, my family doctor, friends, and other acquaintances often demonstrate a lack of understanding related to some types of mental illness. It seems difficult to comprehend how someone who appears to be confident, smart, beautiful, strong, socially acclimated, financially stable, and successful can suffer internally to the degree that requires hospitalization, daily medication, weekly counseling, and academic accommodations. This dichotomy is something that I continue to struggle with throughout my life.

Fortunately, I have learned how to navigate through this confusing space. It was a year and a half before I received an accurate diagnosis for the illness that caused me to check myself into a psychiatric hospital. A year and a half before I was given an explanation for the erratic shifts in my mood or my desperate attempts to avoid abandonment and my attempts to "fix" my highly unstable mood and sense of self. Today, I work to manage, rather than "fix" these insecurities and mood swings that threaten my well-being and ability to survive in a world that often stigmatizes my character.

In this chapter, I use storytelling to create a link between the analytic and the personal as I explore my experiences as a college student living with Borderline Personality Disorder. Through this idea of disease management, I have introduced self-care tools into my daily life in order to successfully navigate college. These integrated self-care tools can also be applied to my social, familial, and work environments. Because of my hospitalization and the continued search for self-identification, I have learned that the structure provided by the use of self-care tools is absolutely necessary for someone diagnosed with Borderline Personality Disorder. One of the greatest lessons learned thus far is that my mental health journey has continuously caused confusion and sometimes disbelief among the people in my life because I may not fit the perceived image of the typical mental health individual. With the help of my self-care tools and strong interpersonal relationships, I have managed to use transparency and disclosure as a way to gain the trust and confidence of my professors, coworkers, family, and bosses so that I can be successful and mentally healthy.

INVISIBLE ILLNESS AND CHRONIC DISEASE

Since the age of thirteen and years leading up to my diagnosis, I have come to view mental health issues as both invisible diseases and chronic illnesses. Others have linked the two terms also, as Susman (1994) understands disability, handicap, and impairment as words that are often interconnected within social scientific research. Within this overlap, disability can be defined as the "loss or abnormality of a psychological, physiological, or anatomical structure or function" that is caused by "chronic illnesses, neuromuscular disease, mental conditions, and cognitive processing problems" (Matthews and Harrington, 2000, p. 405; Susman, 1994, p. 15). These chronic illnesses lead to setbacks, complications, impaired functions, and disabilities (Charmaz 1987). While invisible illness can be interchangeably defined by chronic disease, disability, and handicap, the purpose of this chapter is to focus on the fact that these conditions, both mental and physical, are not innately visible by an observer. As a result, these issues must be studied within the communication field so that the public can better address sufferers and their conditions in a way that allows for self-disclosure, social support, and success, especially among young adults.

As stated previously, research shows that often, we are not aware of chronic medical conditions. According to the 2002 US Census Bureau, about 96 percent of individuals who suffer from a chronic medical condition show no noticeable or outward signs. Similarly, Charmaz (2002) says, chronic illness affects people in ways we do not expect. In fact, "experiencing serious illness challenges prior meanings, ways of living that have been taken for granted, and ways of knowing self; life is now uncertain" (Charmaz, 2002, p. 277). If these experiences are chronicled, sufferers can share their experiences, obstacles, newfound or tainted identities, and fears and uncertainties in a way that increases visibility and challenges dominant ideologies, stereotypes, and stigmas. After all, mental and physical conditions that are not immediately noticeable "influence impression management, and self-disclosure, ultimately impacting health, relationships, and day-to-day functioning" (Harrington and Matthews, 2000, p. 415).

Borderline Personality Disorder (BPD)

Similar to any other invisible illness, Borderline Personality Disorder (BPD) is often subject to stigma and misunderstandings as what we cannot see physically, is often met with disbelief and question. BPD is an illness that is somewhat new to the mental health community and has only recently been more thoroughly explored. According to Bockian, Porr, and Villagram (2002), BPD diagnoses are exponentially growing, causing the need for possible solutions and relief to be of high demand. In fact, nearly 2 percent of Americans have Borderline Personality Disorder with diagnoses being two to three times more likely among young women (Bockian, Porr, and Villagram, 2002).

Research on BPD is relatively new, and the illness is still being defined and redefined. Unlike depression and other mental disorders that can typically be explained by neurobiology, personality disorders like BPD are caused by a combination of biological, psychological, and social factors (Bockian, Porr and Villagram, 2002, p. 7). With such a wide combination of factors, symptoms, and experiences, psychiatrists struggle to diagnose patients with BPD and subsequently, patients often experience incorrect diagnoses.

Borderline personality disorder is characterized by a myriad of attributes including "depression, moodiness, anger, disorganization, anxiety, low self-esteem, rage, feeling that life is meaningless, and feeling that one is unworthy or unlovable" (Bockian, Porr and Villagram, 2002, p. 6). Among other personality disorders, BPD can be diagnosed if at least five symptoms are met within nine specific criteria. These nine criteria have been defined by the *Diagnostic and Statistical Manual of Mental Disorders*, Fourth Edition (DSM-IV) and include avoiding abandonment, unstable and intense relationships, unstable sense of self, impulsive behavior, self-harm or suicidal gestures, unstable mood that lasts through brief periods of time, feelings of emptiness, easily provoked anger, and dissociative symptoms that most commonly proceed stress (Bockian, Porr and Villagram, 2002, p. 7). While many symptoms make up the disorder, BPD can be most easily be defined by the emotional roller coaster experienced by sufferers (Bockian, Porr and Villagram, 2002).

Stigma, Disclosure, and Vulnerability

After the onset of chronic illness, sense of self and identity become vulnerable as "vulnerability derives, in part, from potential disapproval and devaluation" (Charmaz, 2002, p. 277). For those who suffer from a chronic illness and a mental illness like BPD to be specific, stigma is a common battle. In fact, stigma acts as a barrier to self-disclosure with family, friends, and coworkers, which in turn, discourages people from being open about their condition (Cobie're et al., 2013). According to Defenbaugh (2013), "ill individuals often remain socially stigmatized, and those who live with invisible illness must legitimize their ill identity since they infrequently look sick" (p. 159). As a result, those who suffer from an invisible illness have an identity that is viewed as abnormal, unhealthy and is, therefore, socially stigmatized. Goffman (1963) tells us that stigma results in shame, disgrace, and social isolation by virtue of the social devaluation of those who exhibit "Otherness." When aware of one's own "Otherness" the ill individual feels as if he or she does not meet cultural standards and therefore, results in isolation.

Only through disclosure can the chronically ill individual narrate his or her experiences in a way that fights the stigma of mental illness (Corbie're, Samson, Villotti, and Pelletier, 2012). This notion of disclosure can be best understood and utilized through interpersonal contact. Corrigan and Matthews (2003) claim that people who suffer from mental health issues can reduce stigma and negative judgment through openness and disclosure, especially if they make themselves vulnerable in a way that displays confidence, certainty in their diagnosis, and way of life, and strength. A lucid account of experiences that displays the individual overcoming struggle may spark empathy and understanding within the listener or reader. For this reason, the disclosure of stigmatized illnesses is paramount to emotional well-being and furthermore, "likelihood of seeking medical treatment, and family support" (Mellins, Havens, and McCaskill, 2002, p. 455).

Corrigan and Matthews (2003) found that understanding the effects of mental illness and sharing diagnoses lead to significantly improved attitudes. Attitude improvement, building social relationships and developing safe spaces that allow for disclosure without judgment lead to reduced stigma in general. Derlega and Chaikin (1977) explain self-disclosure as "the verbal transmission of information about oneself … [that] contributes to the boundary regulation process" (p. 103). Self-disclosure is particularly important for emotional well-being as Afifi and Steuber (2009) state, "people are likely to reveal the information to relieve their distress… the disclosing of personal information is cathartic in that it allows the body to rid itself of the distress" (p. 146). While little research has been conducted on how to effectively introduce stigmatized topics like mental illness, sharing stories and experiences helps to shed light on the day-to-day struggles those with mental illness endure (Chaudoir and Fisher, 2010). The purpose of this chapter is to explore the lived experiences of someone diagnosed with Borderline Personality Disorder and to discuss the belief that stigma related to mental illness is still present even in well-meaning personal support systems. This chapter acknowledges that one can be a functional, contributing individual within society even when living with an invisible illness. The continued disclosure of my illness to my friends, family, peers, co-workers, and college professors proved to be significantly beneficial for my continued success during my undergraduate studies and ultimately crucial for my every day well-being and future success.

METHOD

I live in a word full of contradiction and only through my own self-reflexive moments that I record and share through the art of storytelling can I make sense of my very confusing flux of emotions. Therefore, the most appropriate way to share my own story is to use the personal voice of autoethnography. I, the researcher, can learn about my own experience with invisible illness through my very own narration while simultaneously sharing my story with others. Autoethnography as a more in depth representation of storytelling is both self-reflexive and self-reflective in the sense that the researcher's story permeates dominant ideologies and cultural stereotypical to share stories and experiences within the mental health community (Crawford, 1996; Berry and Patti, 2015).

Other scholars adhere to the notion as well. Frank (1995) says, "in the reciprocity that is storytelling; the teller offers himself as a guide to the other's self-information" (p. 17–18). In this sense, storytelling provides legitimacy for those who are stigmatized or met with disbelief. My main purpose for sharing this story is to give readers a glimpse into the life and mind of an individual suffering from BPD. Furthermore, in a world that stigmatizes the mentally ill and those with an invisible illness, storytelling and autoethnography allow me to establish myself as a capable and independent human being who, due to my illness, cannot be defined by stereotypes or generalizations thrust upon me. According to Charmaz (2002), it is important to study "what ill people think, feel, and do in their natural settings" in order to truly understand the experience of chronic illness (p. 277). Truly understanding the experience of individuals with chronic illness may contribute to stronger and more empathetic communication. The ability to create a safe space for an individual suffering with mental illness to share their experiences through the use of interpersonal communication and storytelling may lead to an increase in the overall well-being and success in school and within the workforce. What follows is the account of a critical incident and changing point during my mental health journey, which aid in defining who I am as an individual with an invisible, chronic, and most importantly, mental illness.

Part 1: Post-Hospitalization

"Everyone turn to the person sitting to your right," said my professor. "This is the person who you will interview for your profile feature article. The article will talk about what your partner did over winter break." Shit. I spent Christmas day locked away in the mental hospital and then the rest of my break sleeping away the difficult adjustment to new medications. I couldn't even say that I had worked during the break because I was fired from my serving job while admitted in the hospital, after not showing up for my shifts. My partner will think I am crazy. I turned to face him. I had never met him before. At least it's not someone I know, I thought. He was wearing skinny jeans, a beanie, and a band t-shirt. I'm not a fan of generalizations, but perhaps his hipster beard, edgy style, and interest in grungy nineties music made me feel more at ease. After the introductions and small talk he asked, "So, what did you do over break?" I paused for quite some time. I was torn, and fighting with myself over whether I should share the truth or make something up. Flashbacks from the hospital were all I could see.

"I was actually in the mental hospital," I quietly said, waiting and worrying about the reaction I would receive; but he didn't judge me, and he didn't fear me. In fact, he shared a story with me. To my surprise, he had spent a few weeks in the mental hospital during his undergraduate studies at Penn State, too. Moreover, I found out that we had a shared connection. During my first year, I had unknowingly met his fiancé, who had shared a story with the class about her issues with anxiety and depression. I approached her after class to share my common issues because I felt a strong connection to her. Both shared some of the same feelings and experiences that I had, and that gave me an increased desire to be open with them and to pursue friendships. I began to realize that this assignment may not have been the worst way to start a semester after a hospitalization, and in fact, something positive resulted from my disclosure with my new friends, Chris and Mary. Moreover, Ben-Porath (2002), found that in communication among college students, their peers, and their professors can help reduce unnecessary shame associated with treatment.

The next class held yet another surprise for me. The professor stood in front of the class and said, "Now that everyone has a draft of their article, we're going to split up into groups, and read them aloud." Perfect, I thought. I got lucky with sharing my story with Chris who could listen and relate to my experience. However, what were the chances that the entire class would be as understanding? Surely, everyone in the class would now think I'm crazy. Luckily, Chris and I were never in the same group, so I would not have to see anyone's reaction to his paper, or so I thought.

The professor calls for our attention and begins to speak. "Now that everyone has shared their articles with the class, we're going to vote on the two best articles. The author will read his or her article aloud to the class and together, we'll talk about what makes them strong articles and what the writer can do better next time." As luck would have it, Chris's article about me was selected. Based on his slow movement and concerned facial expression, it seemed as if he felt uncomfortable sharing my experience with the entire class. He looked over at me as if to gain my approval before potentially destroying my reputation. I nodded in agreement, and he began revealing my truths. I remember smiling while he read the article. I wanted to appear strong and confident because if I wasn't positive in the eyes of the audience, stigma and negativity might be the result. If I demonstrated that had nothing to hide, then maybe my peers wouldn't think my hospitalization in the mental hospital is any different from a disease or illness that shows physical manifestations in the patient. This was the beginning of how I learned to manage BPD and college, simultaneously.

I do school well. I am a strong writer, prepared for class, and I know how to study. I test well and genuinely want to absorb as much information from my classes as possible. I nod my head, make eye contact, and actively listen when I understand the information. I attribute this to my innate drive, as well as my need to prove that even though I suffer from mental illness, I am a capable, dependable, and intelligent person. However, what I had not expected were the challenges associated with attending college as an individual with Borderline Personality Disorder. Not only was it an unexpected challenge for me, but I also felt that is was something that even my professors could not truly understand. Even so, through disclosure, academic accommodations, and an understanding group of professors, I found a way to navigate the ethos of BPD and academia. I accepted that the combination of college attendance and mental illness wasn't something I would be able to maneuver through without some challenges. However, after my hospitalization, I realized I would need a very specific set of tools and techniques to make it through college and eventually, graduate school.

A regimented structure was key after my hospitalization. I used these techniques to guide me through the rest of my undergraduate studies, which created a smoother transition throughout this process. After self-reflection, I was able to identify the things that caused my symptoms to increase. Stress was one of the biggest triggers to becoming symptomatic, and I began to incorporate some physical activity into my daily routine. I began to tailor my exercise routines based upon the severity of my presenting symptoms; even my exercise routine became extremely specific. On the days that I was overwhelmingly sad and anxious, I went to the gym and ran around the track for as long as I possibly could, sometimes five miles at a time. There were times that I would push myself and continue to run and imagine the sweat as physical beads of stress pouring out of my body alleviating the pain and cleansing me of any negative thoughts. On other days when I felt angry and confused about this illness being a part of my life, I focused on lifting weights, specifically targeting my back and shoulders, where the stress and tension thrived.

In addition to my structured exercise routine, I also maintained employment while in school. This forced me to be more organized and more aware of due dates for assignments and projects. At the beginning of each week, I set aside an allotted amount of time that I used to complete assignments. Each assignment was set to be completed at least three days in advance of the due date. To an outsider, three days might seem extreme, but it was the key to my success. Every single day is unpredictable in my world, and I never know how I am going to react to any incident. If a situation occurs that triggers high levels of anxiety or if my mood suddenly changes negatively, this leads to an unproductive day for me. Therefore, setting deadlines well before due dates t accounts for my possible mood swings or for the days that I am unable to complete an assignment. More importantly, this helped me gain the confidence of my professors because most of my assignments were thorough and handed in on time.

At Penn State, academic accommodations are only administered when documentation from a medical professional is presented to the disabilities coordinator. Presenting this letter from a medical professional was of the utmost importance primarily because it gave me credibility in my claim for accommodations. This key piece of paper legitimized my condition and more so, gave me a starting point from which I could introduce myself, and my condition to each of my professors. Through introductions, disclosure, and openness with each of my professors, I was able to explain my accommodations, my illness, and start to build a rapport. From a conservative approach, some may believe that students should not open up to professors or share personal information. However, if professors reduce the power distance it "create(s) a person-person, friend-friend, or mentor-mentee relationship" (Wang, 2014, p. 77) that students "wanted to get to know better, seek a long-term relationship with, or have as a mentor" (p. 77). This maximized sense of the personal interaction is vital to the development of trust and respect in student-teacher relationships and has proven instrumental in my academic success (Stewart, 2012).

Perhaps the combination of time management, physical exercise, and building relationships with professors has led to my success as a college student with BPD. Or maybe these techniques work because I keep myself so busy that I have very little time to think about my sadness, emptiness, and fears. However, I do feel as though utilizing these tools provide me with the hope and strength that I need to keep me motivated and satisfied with my progress. Most importantly, there existed a huge benefit in building relationships and disclosing my condition with my professors. I was able to use my academic accommodations such as extensions for assignments and rescheduled quizzes and exams. My ability to participate actively in class, produce quality work, spend one-on-one time with professors, and attend class regularly, led to positive interactions with each professor. Nevertheless, even with tools, techniques, and accommodations in place, it is important to remember things do not always go as planned.

Part 2: Instability

"This is bullshit. This event is so unorganized!" I yelled, walking away from the flash mob that I was required to attend as part of my class grade. My professor had worked so hard to make this event happen. Nevertheless, something set me off again, and I walked out on her and the rest of my classmates. Unfortunately, this was not something my accommodations could help mend, so this time, I had to approach the situation differently. During our next class, I received my grade for the flash mob; it was a B-. It was the lowest grade I had ever received. However, what was more concerning was the message my professor left on the back of the paper. "Emily, I was disappointed when I found out that you criticized the team before walking out and missed the entire flash mob. Your actions were very unprofessional."

I fucked up. I don't know what I was thinking. I felt that it wasn't my fault, it was my BPD; but only I knew that. After class, I walked with my professor to her office to address my unprofessional actions at the flash mob. Even though I had given her the academic accommodation letter earlier in the semester, I never truly disclosed how my symptoms, stressors, and emotional struggles affected me. I neglected to share what I was dealing with, so this time I told her. Before I could get the first few words out, the tears fell from my eyes and sank into my jeans, leaving wet spots all over my thighs. My professor reacted with sympathy, handing me a tissue and listening intently. She shared a story with me about a family member who had been dealing with mental health issues, as well. I was comforted knowing that she was able to relate, even though it was through a family member. Moreover, I was so relieved that she understood why I walked out during the flash mob that I do not always have control over what I am feeling or how I react, and that sometimes removing myself from the situation is the only thing that I find helpful. This meeting was the beginning of how I introduced myself to all of my professors. According to Katz, (1957) interpersonal relationships are powerful tools that combat depression and act as social support systems. As I continued to disclose details about my mental health issues, my professors became my social support system. Through my disclosure and openness, I was able to gain the respect and reassurance that I needed from my professors.

Over time, I acknowledged that disclosure with my professors seemed to result in positive responses, so I continued to take classes with those who became part of my social support system. I did not realize at the time that the professor who led the flash mob would play such a huge role in my mental health journey. During my junior year, I was living with my boyfriend and two of our friends. My symptoms were worse than ever, perhaps even worse than before I was hospitalized. Within a three-month period, I had moved out four or five times but would return within an hour or two each time. Some evenings, the fights between my boyfriend and me, often heightened by my BPD symptoms, got so out of control that I would pack my car and drive to my parent's home more than an hour away. One night after a routine fight, my boyfriend left for work, and I decided to pack up all of my belongings. I packed two suitcases full of clothing, my favorite drawings and paintings, my computer, schoolbooks, and anything else of value to me, and drove to my parent's house. This decision consumed hours of my time that could have otherwise been dedicated to my homework or study for an exam the next day I told my roommates that I wasn't coming back, just like I had done all of the previous times, and took off. By the looks of my car, it seemed like I had made a serious decision to leave every time; but within a matter of hours, I was back, smiling as if nothing had gone wrong.

After I had returned one night, I texted my professor to tell her what had happened and how I was feeling. The next day we met to discuss how I could better navigate the situation. I knew something had to change because I wasn't doing my school work; nor was I attending class or my internship regularly. When I did attend class, I wasn't mentally present. A decision was made that I would move in with my professor to regain a sense of stability, return to my school work, and work to get my emotions back to normal. At the time, I had nowhere else to go, I couldn't afford to pay rent elsewhere because I was already locked into a lease with my boyfriend and friends, and commuting from my parent's house seemed to be out the question. Had I not been completely honest with my professor and openly disclosed my struggles with BPD I may never have been able to return to a sense of stability, and consequently, my grades may have suffered. Today, because of my dedication to school despite BPD and disclosure of these struggles with some of the most understanding professors, I achieved a high enough GPA to apply, be accepted, and receive a graduate assistantship to Villanova University, where I study health communication.

Part 3: The Power of Language and Naming

BPD Diagnosis and Linguistic Relativity

"Have you ever heard of Borderline Personality Disorder?" Dr. Mike asked me. "Not Multiple Personality Disorder," he added. "It's not even similar to that. It's more like Bipolar Disorder, which I see you have been diagnosed with after your hospitalization." The unfamiliar condition sounded serious, but I was not afraid of the potential diagnosis. In fact, I was excited to learn about it. I craved an understanding of what I was going through, and I craved a sense of identity. As Dr. Mike listed off the criteria for the diagnosis, my excitement grew. "That's me!" I said. My isolating, erratic, and impulsive decisions, sense of hopelessness, anxiety, unstable sense of self, and fear of abandonment all seemed to come together under this umbrella term called Borderline Personality Disorder. Throughout my entire adolescent life, I was diagnosed based on these individual symptoms. By the time, I was nineteen, I had been diagnosed with Major Depressive Disorder, General Anxiety Disorder, and Bipolar Disorder; but none of these diagnoses encompassed all of the symptoms that I was experiencing. Now that I found a word that described all of my symptoms, I would be able to develop a stronger identity and finally fit into a specific group. I was finally part of something greater than I was, and with this diagnosis, I could help other people like myself. Linguistic relativity helps to make sense of this phenomenon.

My experiences suggest that language heavily influences my everyday perceptions. Linguistic relativity, theorized by Sapir-Whorf, helps me make sense of both an objective and social reality. Sapir-Whorf explained how the power of naming helps make sense of the world around us. What's more, they said that until we understand something linguistically, humans can't talk about it (Fritch, Ice, and Palczewski, 2012). For this reason, until something has been named, people are unable to understand the phenomenon or determine if the situation or idea is for a good cause. In this case, I use the term

Borderline Personality Disorder to make sense of my condition so that I can better understand why I behave the way I do and how I can adjust my behavior to navigate this serious mental health condition. Because this term has been used to make sense of a fairly new mental health condition, various perceptions of BPD have emerged.

While it may not be intentional, mass communication can be considered a culprit for providing representations that communicate the misrecognition of those who are mentally ill. It may be difficult for those in society to recognize or identify with illnesses that are not visible; unfortunately, they cannot "see" the hurt or pain present on the inside. Mental health issues can be paralyzing and painful conditions that should be addressed and recognized as legitimate illnesses. It is also important that individuals learn to see the person, not the condition or illness because people identify with their condition; while others do not. As these perceptions emerge and we begin to make sense of mental illness linguistically, it is important to help people understand the importance of interpersonal relationships, disclosures, and transparency in mental health remission. In this sense, this research aims to understand the experiences and lifestyle associated with mental health and works to renegotiate the term Borderline Personality Disorder so that the health condition is no longer misrepresented. Moreover, I want this work to act as a self-care guide for college students who are burdened with mental illness while trying to survive college.

CONCLUSION

As a student with BPD who still struggles with mental health issues, I have learned a great deal about myself including how my mind works, and how I can be the most productive version of myself during my undergraduate studies. I recognize my disability and work to dismantle its incredibly confusing and behavioral consequences every single day. It is a constant battle for me daily. While many people in my life refuse to reconcile with the fact that I am chronically and mentally ill, it is important to remember that illness is not something that is always observable physically or outwardly. I chose to embrace my diagnosis of Borderline Personality Disorder in a way that has always left the people in my life confused. They have always stated that I do not fit the perceived image of an individual with mental health issues. Ultimately, this misrecognition may delegitimize the ill individual's condition. To avoid such tension, I employed a very specific set of tools as a means of transcending illness. While self-care tools did not always prevent symptoms from increasing, they provided structure during particularly unstable days.

Through the art of ethnography, I used storytelling to link the personal and analytical, and in doing so, separated myself from my experiences so that

I could better examine my story. As Frank (2012) explains, creating distance "between the narrator and the protagonist" allows the storyteller to use vulnerability as a form of strength and courage (p. 48). Self-disclosure has led to strength and growth within my life, which has ultimately enabled me equal access to higher education. Above all, personal disclosure related to my mental illness shared with my professors and peers has created an environment of trust and acceptance that I continued to build upon and strengthen during my college career.

REFERENCES

Afifi, A., and Steuber, K. (2009). "The revelation risk model (RRM): Factors that predict the revelation of secrets and the strategies used to reveal them." *Communication Monographs*, 76, 144–176.

Ben-Porath. (2002). "Receive Psychotherapy: An Interaction Between Help-seeking Behavior and the Presence of Depression." *Journal of Social and Clinical Psychology. 21(4).* Doi 10.1521/jscp.21.4.400.22594

Berry, K., and Patti, C. (2015). "Lost in narration: Applying autoethnography." *Journal of Applied Communication Research. 43(2).* doi:10.1080/00909882.2015.1019548

Chaudoir, S. R., and Fisher, J. D. (2010). "The disclosure process model: Understanding disclosure decision-making and post-disclosure outcomes among people with a concealable stigmatized identity." *Psychological Bulletin*, 136(2), 236–256. doi:10.1037=a0018193

Corbie`re, M., Samson, E., Villotti, P., and Pelletier, J. (2012). "Strategies to fight stigma toward people with mental disorders: Perspectives from different stakeholders." *Scientific World Journal*, 2012, 1–10. doi:10.1100=2012=516358

Crawford, L. (1996). "Personal ethnography." *Communication Monographs,* 63, 158–170. doi :101080/03637759609376384

Defenbaugh, N. L. (2013). "Revealing and Concealing Ill Identity: A Performance Narrative of IBD Disclosure." *Health Communication*, *28*(2), 159–169. doi:10.1080/10410236.2012.666712

Derlega, V. J., and Chaikin, A. L. (1977). "Privacy and self-disclosure in social relationships." *Journal of Social Issues,* 33, 102–115.

Frank, A. W. (1995). *The wounded storyteller: Body, illness, and ethics.* Chicago: University of Chicago Press.

Frank, A. W. (2012). *Practicing Dialogical Narrative Analysis.*

Fritch, J., Ice, R., Palczewski, C.H. (2012). *Rhetoric and Civic Life.* State College, PA: Strata Publishing, Inc.

Goffman, E. (1963). *Stigma: Notes on the Management of Spoiled Identity.* Englewood Cliffs, NJ: Prentice-Hall

Higgins, M. A. (2000, November). "Protecting the public's privacy by mediating disclosures about disability." Paper Presented at the National Communication Association Conference, Seattle, WA.

Holmes, M. S. (2015). "Embodied Storytellers: Disability Studies and Medical Humanities." *Hastings Center Report*, *45*(2), 11–15. doi:10.1002/hast.426

Katz, E. (1957). "The two-step flow of communication: An up-to-date report on a hypothesis." *Public Opinion Quarterly, 21,* 61–78.

Matthews, C. K., and Harrington, N. G. (2000). "Invisible disability." In D. O. Braithwaite & T. L. Thomspon (Eds.), *Handbook of communication and people with disabilities: Research and application* (pp. 405–421). Mahwah, NJ: Lawrence Erlbaum Associates, Inc.

Mellins, C. A., Havens, J. F., and McCaskill, E. O. (2002). "Mental health, substance use and disclosure are significantly associated with the medical treatment adherence of HIV-infected mothers." *Psychology, Health & Medicine*, 7(4), 451–460.

Quinlan, M. M. (2014). "Invisible disabilities." In T. L. Thompson (Ed.), *Encyclopedia of health communication* (pp. 754–755). Thousand Oaks, CA: Sage. Ward, B. W. (2012).

Stewart, J. (Ed.). (2012). *Bridges not walls: A book about interpersonal communication* (11th ed.). New York, NY: McGraw-Hill.

Susman, J. (1994). "Disability, stigma and deviance." *Social Science and Medicine*, 38, 15–22.

US Census Bureau. (2002). *Americans with Disabilities.* Retrieved from January 17, 2017, from https://www.census.gov/prod/2006pubs/p70–107.pdf

Van Maanen, J. (2011). *Tales of the field: On writing ethnography.* Chicago: University of Chicago Press.

Wang, T. R. (2014). "Formational Turning Points in the Transition to College: Understanding How Communication Events Shape First-Generation Students' Pedagogical and Interpersonal Relationships With Their College Teachers." *Communication Education*, *63*(1), 63–82. doi:10.1080/03634523.2013.841970\

Chapter Five

An Unexpected Road to Discovery

Finding One's Self in the Midst of Uncertainty

Launick Saint-Fort

It was the end of a strenuous yet, unfruitful research week in the laboratory. As usual, I was overwhelmed with disappointment. I had dedicated countless hours to my experiments with no plausible outcome to show—the "oh so" inevitable fate of a research fellow might I say. This feeling of discontent had become common, and I desired to break free from the pessimism. Though frustrated, I decided to do my good deed for the week by donating blood. Blood donation had always been of great significance to my family because my brother was diagnosed with a red blood cell disorder, Sickle-Cell Anemia during childhood. My brother has always relied on the generosity of donors for his monthly blood transfusions. As a family, we recognized the importance of donating blood and wanted to contribute to this cause. I arrived at the blood blank and waited for the nurse to call my name. My fear of needles led to a state of mild panic and anxiety. The thought of a 17-gauge needle piercing through my veins was unsettling to say the least, but I reminded myself that this was a necessary sacrifice for a much bigger cause.

My name was called and I began taking noticeably deep breaths. Attempting to ignore puzzling stares I nervously walked to my donation station. In my mind, I was sure they were finding it difficult to believe that an adult could be so fearful of needles. To my relief, the nurse managed to find my vein on the first try; a great feat for someone with deep veins. My good deed for the week was accomplished; I could go home and plan for the weekend ahead.

I packed my things, left the clinic and headed to the busy Metro train station, but quickly realized something was wrong. My head felt heavy, my heart was racing, I was losing control of my body but I kept on walking.

Dizzy and rapidly becoming unaware of my surroundings I managed to reach the escalator. It seemed like the steepest escalator I had ever encountered.

Inquiries of concerned citizens surround me as I struggled to lower myself on the steps. A Good Samaritan attended to me while I waited for the ambulance, as hurried Metro riders rushed to their arriving trains.

It was my first time in an ambulance and to my dismay, it was rather calm, nothing like the movies—no sirens, no speeding through traffic, and no overzealous paramedics. My symptoms must not have been alarming I supposed; an assertion that was later confirmed by the emergency room doctor. I was sent home and things went back to normal. I assumed this mishap was an isolated incident but as the days went by, it was clear to me that the battle had not yet ended.

I spent the next few weeks baffled over the reasons why walking half a mile suddenly felt like a marathon and my activities of daily living were no longer a breeze. I tried tirelessly to convince my doctors that my symptoms were not figments of my imagination, nevertheless, they insisted that my illness was no mystery but likely a case of depression and/ or anxiety. In my heart, I knew that this prognosis could not entirely justify my ailments and subsequently found myself caving into a deep state of stasis and desperation. I was a medical enigma and no one could pinpoint the underlying cause of my symptoms. I wondered if they were a manifestation of anxiety or something more profound. Illness is familiar territory for someone like me; born destitute in Haiti, a fourth world nation devastated by poverty, disease, natural disasters, political instability, violence, and illiteracy. As a child, I suffered from an array of childhood diseases that were easily preventable through vaccination and almost unheard of in the developed world. However, those days of sorrow and hopelessness ended once I arrived in the United States on December 6, 1999.

Snow and sub-zero degree temperatures greeted me as I landed in the Big Apple, New York City. I had never experienced the cold before. How would I survive life in what felt like a refrigerator? I could not fathom how anyone could live in such conditions after all, I was born on a tropical island surrounded by oceans and palm trees. I was a foreigner in a place where the language was distant and the people as diverse as can be; nonetheless, I cheered to new beginnings. The American dream I yearned for my entire childhood was no longer a figment of my imagination. I was in the land of the brave and the free and anything was possible. Determined not to take for granted this invaluable opportunity, I applied myself to the best of my abilities and eventually became a first-generation college graduate. The vicious cycle seen much too often in my family was finally broken and I was proud to carry the torch and lead the way.

In college, I was a non-traditional student and maintained multiple jobs during my studies; nevertheless, I somehow managed to excel academically as a biochemistry major. Walking across the stage to accept my degree and shaking the chancellor's hands, signified years of struggle and defying the odds. I remembered the countless times I was told that my goals were much too ambitious and that I was reaching for the unattainable and yet, here I was, concluding my journey as an undergrad and looking forward to a prestigious fellowship. As a fellow, my focus was research to assist with the eradication of neglected tropical diseases. I looked forward to studying for my GRE exam and applying to graduate school. It all seemed like a fairy tale. I had slayed the evil queen, gained control of my kingdom, and would live happily after. No one could stop me, not today, not tomorrow. Little did I know, the evil queen and her henchmen were waiting in the shadows with another unprecedented hurdle; postural orthostatic tachycardia syndrome.

Postural orthostatic tachycardia syndrome (POTS) is an ambiguous clinical syndrome indicated by a supine-to-standing heart rate increase in the absence of postural hypotension (Johnson et al., 2010). POTS is a multiplexed disorder with an array of symptoms that include neuropathic pain, poor sleep efficiency, chronic fatigue, headaches, palpitations, tremors, gastrointestinal disturbance, facial flushing, and orthostatic symptoms like dizziness, lightheadedness, and syncope (Ojha, Chelimsky, and Chelimsky, 2011). Overall, this poorly understood condition manifests in young, well-educated women, like myself but can occur in both genders at any age.

POTS poses many challenges for physicians and patients alike because of its varying etiology and co-morbid diagnoses. Without approved US Food and Drug Administration medications for the treatment of POTS, physicians may resort to prescribing off-label medications. However, many medications used to treat co-morbid conditions may exacerbate POTS symptoms and offer little relief to patients under current treatment regimens for the syndrome (Garland, Celedonio, and Raj, 2015).

The effect on the quality of life in these patients can be mild with minor disruptions in daily activities or severe and affecting activities of daily living such as eating or showering. Physical functioning, bodily pain, general health, and social functioning are significantly impaired in those with POTS (Bruce et al., 2016). A quarter of those suffering with POTS are estimated to be disabled and unable to work or to attend school. Furthermore, the severity of orthostatic intolerance symptoms (e.g., lightheadedness, brain fog, and palpitations) can lead to both depression and diminished quality of life in POTS patients (Benrud-Larson et al., 2002). The quality of life in POTS patients is comparable to those with rheumatoid arthritis, end-stage renal disease, congestive heart failure, and chronic obstructive pulmonary disease (Bruce et al., 2016).

I had never heard of this rare disorder before and given my luck, of course I would be the one to contribute to the two hundred thousand or so US cases per year. Surely a diagnosis would ease my woes and pave the way for times devoid of doubt and unwarranted cynicism. I would return to my usual practice of overcoming the never-ending impediments of my life and work to become a fearsome chemist in six-inch heels and bold red lips; an auspicious outlook that would later prove to be a half-truth. My experiences with illness were restricted to my days as a prepubescent child in Haiti, thus the impact of illness on life as an adult in America was a predicament I had not yet encountered. This lack of familiarity would ultimately become grounds for many false assumptions pertaining to my emotional response to this newfound illness.

Response to medical illness can be attributed to a person's perception of the illness and a diagnosis can trigger panic, depression, or anger (Gazzola and Muskin, 2003). In truth, my condition rekindled my overwhelming frustrations with doctors who seemed apathetic to my struggles because according to them, I was armed with the optimism of youth. I became overly agitated with their nonchalant approach and felt as though I was slowly losing my mind. I was in severe pain, exasperated and wanted to bang my head against the walls every time I heard the words "you're young, you'll be fine". As a matter of fact, it was even suggested that my pain was more psychological than physiological, which nearly drove me to the point of insanity. Were these doctors discounting my agony? Perhaps there was validity to their claim.

In fact, research and clinical experience associated with pain indicate that the correlation between the amount of tissue damage and the degree of discomfort or functional disability reported by the patient is indeterminate.

> The nature of the pain and its underlying physiological factors affect the course from acute pain to chronic pain to functional disability. Yet for many, and perhaps most, of those who go through this process, psychosocial factors are inextricably intertwined with physiological change and may even be primary (Osterweis, Kleinman, and Mechanic, 1987, p. 1).

"A crucial premise in the study of illness behavior is that illness, as well as the illness experience, are shaped by psychological, social, and cultural factors irrespective of the genetic, physiological, or other biological bases of disease" (Osterweis et al., 1987, p.1). Thus, the perception of illness is a key factor when analyzing how patients cope with chronic illness.

Correspondingly, patients often exhibit adaptations mirroring their personality traits and I was no different (Falcone and Franco, 2010). Considering my incessant need to triumph, the possibility of being limited by my condition was inconceivable. As expected, the physicians did not recognize this prominent attribute of mine and therefore, were unable to customize a plan of care unique to not only my medical condition, but to me as a person. The failure of my physicians to identify and appropriately respond to these innate behavioral patterns made me feel misunderstood and quite frankly, mistreated. "Recognizing these traits and appropriate responses to them by healthcare personnel increase the likelihood that patients will respond optimally to care management" (Groves and Muskin, 2005, p. 70).

As the disparity between what I perceived to be individualized care as opposed to standard medicine became apparent, I thought it best to utilize my skills as a researcher to become an active participant in overcoming my illness. Accordingly, my mission was to delve into research articles to better understand my ailment and the treatment options available; particularly non-medicinal alternatives. This strategy was paired with visiting forums of current and past sufferers of POTS to explore various coping mechanisms that may be implemented in my journey to better health. Having a sense of control and direction as a resilient female were perhaps the most useful methods in coping with my symptoms. Ultimately, having control over one's health and well-being results to greater harmony with health care providers to achieve rehabilitation (Falcone, and Franco, 2010).

Coping styles differ among patients and are often predominant defenses that protect one from distress (Falcone and Franco, 2010). A hierarchical organization of defenses were suggested by Vaillant's *Ego Mechanism of Defense: A Guide for Clinicians and Researchers* ranging from psychotic to immature, neurotic and mature.

> Studies of the relation between defenses and coping styles indicate that high-functioning persons use predominantly mature and neurotic defenses, whereas less-resilient persons, generally those with personality disorders—exhibit more primitive (immature and psychotic) defense mechanisms. Examples of defense mechanisms include suppression (mature), repression (neurotic), passive-aggressive behavior (immature), and denial (psychotic) (Vaillant, 1992, p. 29)

It is safe to say that my defenses were an admix of the many described by Vaillant. To my surprise, my initial response was one of significant denial an unforeseeable turn of events for a high-functioning person such as myself. Though my last visit to the doctors was years prior, I was adamant that I was in good health and that this occurrence was undeniably transient. At times, this denial was accompanied by a display of passive-aggressive behavior leading to interpersonal conflicts between my physicians and myself. In due course, I began to suppress my fears as they proved to be the greatest barrier to improving my health.

"Personality, chronic pain, and illness behavior interact in complex ways that are not fully understood" (Osterweis et al., 1987, p. 5). The bridge between these three elements was previously non-existent in my world as I had become accustomed to pain and always dismissed the possibility that my pain may be the cause of a more significant issue. Charade had become the norm as it was easier to move forward through life unaware of my reality.

I believed this mentality to have been the precursor to my diagnosis and in the end, I was overwhelmed with guilt. Surely, if I had been more proactive about determining the root of my pain, all of this could have been prevented. Was this the consequence of self-neglect or simply serendipity? I may never know but the constant battle between succumbing to one's circumstances or taking action as derivatives of sociocultural factors were apparent.

The role of mistrust in the African American medical care experience is one of great historical perspective and is deeply embedded in black communities (Eiser and Ellis, 2007). This abundance of skepticism stems from the unavailability and/or lack of quality health care afforded to African Americans throughout America's history. Medically related discrimination and segregation were conventional and led to the infamous Public Health Service-sponsored experiment involving African Americans—the Tuskegee syphilis study (Rosenberg, 1987). In this study, researchers did not inform of the patients about the experiment; treatment was withheld without the patients' knowledge (The Belmont Report, 1979).

Today, the effects of the study, as well as numerous negative clinical research experiences linger in African American communities, further perpetuating wariness in the American health care system (Eiser and Ellis, 2007). Given these dark and unsolicited incidences among others, it is not surprising that I, a black woman in America, would normalize pain as justification to not seek medical care. This mentality, though valid to some extent; continues to be a significant component of the health disparities seen between black and white Americans.

Prior to my illness, I was completely unaware of my medical history and was dumbfounded whenever my doctors inquired about past medical procedures and examinations. I believed visits to a gynecologist were solely for sexually active women, physical exams, only if required for employment and when life happens, one would visit the emergency room. I refrained from smoking, drinking, excessive partying, and made relatively good choices. The need to see a doctor did not feel like a necessity. I was in complete denial and deemed myself as invincible. These convictions were a heavy burden for my doctors as they constructed my medical dossier to better understand the origins of my condition.

Needless to say, I was subjected to numerous laboratory tests, which only amplified my angst. Although these recurring trips to the doctors' offices were very frustrating, they ultimately revealed medical disorders previously unknown to me. I was diagnosed with anemia and, asthma along with a host of other disorders. While these revelations were quite surprising, the most alarming of them all was my diagnosis with depression. I remember being asked simple questions such as: do you have little interest or pleasure in doing things? Any trouble falling or staying asleep? Do you feel down, depressed or hopeless? The doctor was able to ask these questions without disclosing their purpose because had she informed me that the interrogation was to examine my mental health, I am certain that I would not have answered the questions truthfully.

In African American communities, mental health is a topic that is widely misconstrued and rarely discussed. This lack of awareness leads many African Americans to believe that experiencing challenges in mental health issues are a sign of personal weakness or punishment from God; thus such conditions are associated with shame and stigma. Furthermore, Dr. Jane Taylor, a psychiatrist, implies a cultural component in which providers are often culturally insensitive to the plight of African Americans. Although I am Haitian born, my brown body and lived experiences are culturally similar to those of American born blacks. "There are some health care providers who assume that…strife in black people or having a difficult time are what's to be expected," said Dr. Taylor. "…In some cases they may normalize what may be a traumatic reaction." (Hamm, 2012, para. 6).

Undoubtedly, my depression was a psychological response to the debilitating effects of POTS. I was too sick to work and could barely stand on my feet without feeling like I would fall, hit my head and incur a traumatic brain injury. This fear forced me to be a prisoner in my own home. I would spend days contemplating all the things I wanted to do, but was physically unable to accomplish. The thought of being "stuck" was too much to bare and I became angry with life. I believed this to be the end of my journey to success. "This cannot be how it all ends," I said to myself. "I was made from the fire". This brought forth a recollection of memories from my disconsolate childhood on an impoverished island.

My experiences as an underprivileged child in Haiti created great dependence on the mercy of others. These experiences were enough to make anyone with the slightest bit of benevolence cry; yet, I remained intact. How could sickness, particularly one that is non-life threatening pose such a significant threat to my conquest? Many people fall ill and the world never ceases to revolve. I could have been one of the 250,000 casualties of Haiti's 2010 devastating earthquake, but I was not. I could have been a young woman back home with no prospects and no avenues for better life, but I was not.

The opportunities offered to me in America could not be taken for granted and these constant reminders of what life "could have been" gave me the will to move on; even at my weakest moments. Nevertheless, my will to move on was challenged by the unpredictability and potentially debilitating impact of POTS. Indeed, this diagnosis triggered my unexpected ordeal with depression.

"Uncertainty is a common component of the illness experience and can increase the burden of managing chronic illness" (Reich, Johnson, Zautra, and Davis, 2006, p. 308). Illness uncertainty is often described as a "cognitive stressor, a sense of loss of control, and a perception about one's illness that changes over time" (Reich et al., 2006, p. 309). Nonetheless, the most cohesive definition of illness uncertainty is "the inability to determine the meaning of illness-related events (that) occurs in situations where the decision-maker is unable to assign definite values to objects and events and/or is unable to accurately predict outcomes because sufficient cues are lacking" (Mishel, Hostetter, King, and Graham, 1984, p. 291).

POTS is unpredictable. One day I am strong enough to walk out of the house and the next, I can barely get out of bed. Mornings were exceptionally difficult due to excessive pain from costochondritis, chronic fatigue from insomnia and heart palpitations from being in a postural position during the night. The impact of my illness on my training as a fellow could not be ignored. I began to contemplate the options between continuing my fellowship and going back home to Pennsylvania. I could no longer withstand the pressures of being in a lab and working irregular hours.

My health became my priority and in this new realm of mine, reality preceded passion. Through the struggle I reminded myself that I was not one to cower and run when life gets tough—I examine the problem and find solutions. I refused to allow my illness to diminish my hard work and perseverance. I reminded myself of where I aspired to be in ten years. This simple, yet critical query would inadvertently lead to the beginning of my road to discovery of living with and managing this illness.

The first step would require the courage to be open and reach out to my mentors for guidance. It was clear to my mentors that I was lost and frightened and as good mentors they provided a listening ear for my concerns. The care-seeking mentality can be seen from an evolutionary perspective, which draws us to those who can provide support and resources in times of need (Hermanto, Zuroff, Kelly, and Leybman, 2017).

Other researchers assert that:

> Prior work has found that those with high quality or quantity of social networks have a decreased risk of mortality in comparison to those who have low quantity or quality of social relationships, even after statistically controlling for baseline health status. In fact, social isolation itself was identified as an independent major risk factor for all-cause mortality. (Reblin and Uchino, 2008, p. 201)

Seeking support from others was not an easy task. I have always thought of myself as a warrior; strong and able to fight my battles alone. The idea of asking for help seemed cowardly. I began to wonder if the luxuries of being an American had made me weak. I needed to "get back up and fight as usual" because this too, shall pass. But this battle, I could not win on my own. I needed a few good soldiers by my side and they came in the form of family members, close friends, supervisors and to my surprise, counselors.

At first, my bias toward counseling was so erroneous that I am now embarrassed to allude to these past impressions. In my mind, counseling was for those faced with addiction and psychological ailments. Each time my doctor would suggest the idea of counseling, I retaliated with a score of rebuttals. I would envision myself laying on a couch with the counselor sitting across from me with legs crossed, a pen and paper, probing me to tell him/her what troubled me. I thought this scenario to be ludicrous. It was hard to imagine how a stranger, with no background knowledge of who I was, could help me to combat my illness. I felt that I would rather suffer in silence than to subject myself to such nonsense.

Health care providers and society sometimes dismiss the psychological impact of illness in general. Coping with chronic illness involves managing both the physiologic changes that occur as well as the complex outcomes that result as a consequence of illness (Aguilar, 1997). The psychological implications of my illness revealed themselves in the ways I interacted with others. I spent most of my days in confinement. When I did leave my apartment, I could not relinquish the thought of rushing home to lie down. I refused to attend social events and the drive to partake in my beloved pastimes dissipated into thin air. My insomnia worsened and my mood fluctuated. I was desperate for an intervention and after much consideration, decided that counseling was worth a try.

There was something invigorating about sharing my plight with someone without the fear of judgment or reprisal. Being directed to various illness related resources helped me to adjust my lifestyle to better accommodate my illness. These new adjustments not only alleviated my depression, and insomnia; but also my chronic pain. Although the heart palpitations and shortness of breath are usually present, they are now more manageable. My disdain for psychotherapy departed and counseling had become an important tool in coping with my illness.

Perhaps the most fascinating revelation of dealing with my condition was the sudden change of heart to pursue a career in medicine. This came as surprise to not only myself, but to everyone who has followed my journey in college. I believed I was destined to be a chemist and to become a pioneer in the development of diagnostic devices for field detection of diseases in areas where resources are scarce. I was good at chemistry and relished in the idea of becoming a black female chemist at the forefront of microfluidic innovations.

For years, I lived life on overdrive and seldom took the time to consider my quality of life. I needed a reality check and this illness was exactly that. It compelled me to re-assess my values and whether my current choice of career would allow me to live the fulfilling and purposeful life that I've always dreamed about. It did not. I realized that the culture of a lab did not suit my extroverted personality. I was deprived of the meaningful human interactions that I desired and therefore felt disconnected from the world. It was humbling to be a part of the research community, but the effect of my research on humanity was unclear. The idea that my livelihood as a scientist was contingent upon publications in revered scientific journals was uninspiring. My undergraduate education had given me a false representation of life as a researcher,. As an undergraduate researcher, I was not subjected to ten hour days in the lab nor experienced fierce competition between my lab mates and I. I was not prepared for life as a researcher but thankfully, my illness allowed me the opportunity be more objective during my training as a fellow while I explored alternate career paths.

The importance of scientific inquiry for the advancement of human-kind is one that cannot be disputed. As a researcher, I failed to see the direct impact on the people whose clinical samples I was investigating. The probability that my findings would lead to inconclusive results or the need for further scientific studies that would transpire years after the initial inquiry was disheartening. Nevertheless, my love for science persisted and I was on a mission to find a profession that would allow me to pair my passion for science with my desire to help others live longer and healthier lives. Living with an invisible illness further reinforced the discovery that a career in medicine was the right path.

Most importantly, this unforeseen experience with illness has been instrumental in lifting the veil that I proudly wore for so long. This veil—a combination of my perceived invulnerability and tenacity—did nothing but impair my perception of reality. It unearthed just how dangerous the fear of the unknown could be. The fear of not knowing what my future with POTS entailed, dominated the primary experiences with my illness, and I allowed this fear to cripple me in more ways than one.

> One great enemy we must all endeavor to fear is not conquering. Fear can cripple purpose and purposeful life. Fear asks question we must fear. Fear makes vision a nightmare. One must always cross the barrier of fear to get to the great city of true purposefulness. A great number of us who are unable to live to accomplish the true reason for our existence on earth are unable to cross the barrier of fear in the first place. (Ernest Agyemang Yeboah cited in Dalloh, 2016, para. 23)

I was petrified of watching my hopes and dreams fade into the shadows and finding myself enclosed within the invisible box that was designed for poor women of color. I was afraid of disappointing those who willingly dedicated their time and efforts in my expedition to a more purposeful life. To me, succeeding in life was the best gift that I could give them for their endless support. But as I came to accept my illness, I realized that fear had never held such significance in my life. Before my illness much of my future was undetermined, yet I continued to face my hurdles without fear. Why was I so inclined to distinguish illness as a distinct entity? Illness is just one of the many facets of life that most of us, at some point in time, will encounter. Rather than being stricken with fear, it would be beneficial to learn to find comfort in discovering new perspectives and reconstructing a new self.

In the end, I not only found freedom in my illness but also a new self; one who has finally mastered the art of self-compassion. Instead of mercilessly judging and criticizing myself for various inadequacies or shortcomings, I have learned to be kind and understanding when confronted with personal failings. I have accepted that asking for help is not a display of weakness, but rather an acknowledgement that even the strongest of us sometimes need a shoulder to lean on. I often take time to self-reflect in areas of happiness, contentment, and my fulfillment toward my purpose in life. I also remind myself that life is more than just a list of accolades and recognitions that do not define who I truly am.

Like illness, life, in its entirety, is uncertain and this uncertainty is integral in my continuous efforts to be a better self. Not knowing what tomorrow brings opens my minds to new possibilities and a world that does not exist solely in my dreams. I strive to continue on this road to discovery because finding one's self does not occur in one isolated moment. It materializes little by little until we feel complete. The sooner we embark on this journey, the brighter the light will be at the end of the tunnel. My faith in myself has been restored and I can say with the utmost conviction that the best has yet to come.

REFERENCES

"African American mental health." (n.d.). *National Alliance on Mental Illness*. Retrieved from https://www.nami.org/Find-Support/Diverse-Communities/African-Americans

Aguilar, N. (1997). "Counseling the patient with chronic illness: Strategies for the health care provider." *Journal of the American Academy of Nurse Practitioners*, *9*(4), 171–175.

The Belmont Report: Ethical Principles and Guidelines for the Protection of Human Subjects of Research. (1979). Retrieved from https://videocast.nih.gov/pdf/ohrp_appendix_belmont_report_vol_1.pdf

Benrud-Larson, L. M., Dewar, M. S., Sandroni, P., Rummans, T. A., Haythornthwaite, J. A., Low, P. A. (2002). "Quality of life in patients with postural orthostatic tachycardia syndrome." *Mayo Clinic Proceedings*, *77*(6), 531–537.

Bruce, B. K., Harrison, T. E., Bee, S. M., Luedtke, C. A., Porter, C.-B. J., Fischer, P. R., Hayes S. E., Allman, D. A., Ale, C. M., and Weiss, K. E. (2016). "Improvement in functioning and psychological distress in adolescents with postural orthostatic tachycardia syndrome following interdisciplinary treatment." *Clinical Pediatrics*, *55*(14), 1300–304.

Dalloh, A. (2016). "Generation 2063 schools and education program." *AU-Watch*. Retrieved from http://dev.marijawo.com/au-watch.org/?q=agenda-2063/generation-2063-schools-and-education-program

Eiser, A. R., and Ellis, G. (2007). "Viewpoint: Cultural competence and the African American experience with health care: The case for specific content in cross-cultural education." *Academic Medicine*, *82*(2), 176–83.

Falcone, T., and Franco, K. N. (2010). "Coping with chronic medical illness." In William D. Carey (Ed.), *Current Clinical Medicine* (2nd ed.) (pp. 1013–1016).

Garland, E. M., Celedonio, J. E., and Raj, S. R. (2015). "Postural Tachycardia Syndrome: Beyond orthostatic intolerance." *Current neurology and neuroscience reports*, *15*(9), 60.

Gazzola, L. R. A., and Muskin, P. R. (2003). "The impact of stress and the objectives of psychosocial interventions." In: L. A. Schein, H. S. Bernard, H. I. Spitz, and P. R. Muskin (Eds.), *Psychosocial treatment for medical conditions: Principles and techniques*. (pp. 373–406). New York, NY: Brunner-Routledge.

Groves, M., and Muskin, P. (2005). "Psychological responses to illness." In: J. L. Levenson (Ed.), *The American psychiatric publishing textbook of psychosomatic medicine* (pp. 68–88). Washington, DC: American Psychiatric Association.

Hamm, N. (2012, October 1). "Black folks and mental health: Why do we suffer in silence?" *Ebony*. Retrieved from http://www.ebony.com/wellness-empowerment/black-folks-and-mental-health-610#axzz4gVnUF9Jf

Hermanto, N., Zuroff, D. C., Kelly, A. C., Leybman, M. J. (2017). "Receiving support, giving support, and self-reassurance: A daily diary test of social mentality theory." *Personality and Individual Differences*, *107*, 37–42.

Johnson, J. N., Mack, K. J., Kuntz, N. L., Brands, C. K., Porter, C. J., and Fisher, P. R. (2010). "Postural orthostatic tachycardia syndrome: A clinical review." *Pediatric Neurology*, *42*(2), 77–85.

Mishel, M. H., Hostetter, T., King, B., and Graham, V. (1984). "Predictors of psychosocial adjustment in patients newly diagnosed with gynecological cancer." *Cancer Nursing*, *7*(4), 291–299.

Ojha, A., Chelimsky, T. C., and Chelimsky, G. (2011). "Comorbidities in pediatric patients with postural orthostatic tachycardia syndrome." *Journal of Pediatrics, 158*(1), 20–23.

Osterweis, M., Kleinman, A., and Mechanic, D. (1987). *Pain and disability: Clinical, behavioral, and public policy perspectives*. Washington, DC: National Academic Press.

Reblin, M., and Uchino, B. N. (2008). "Social and emotional support and its implication for health." *Current Opinion in Psychiatry*, *21*(2), 201–205.

Reich, J. W., Johnson, L. M., Zautra, A. J., and Davis, M. C. (2006). "Uncertainty of illness relationships with mental health and coping processes in Fibromyalgia patients." *Journal of Behavioral Medicine*, *29*(4), 307–316.

Rosenberg, C. E. (1987). *The care of strangers*. New York, NY: Basic Books.

Vaillant, G. E. (1992). *Ego mechanisms of defense: A guide for clinicians and researchers*. Washington, DC: American Psychiatric Association.

Chapter Six

When Lifestage Matters

A Narrative Account of a Pregnancy-Related Invisible Illness

Eletra S. Gilchrist-Petty

Illnesses can come in many forms—some are visible, while others are invisible and more understated. Some illnesses are not only invisible but only occur during certain stages of life. As long as you are not in a lifestage that ignites the illness, you can live symptom-free and virtually have what is typically defined, as a normal life. This chapter uses personal narrative as a methodology to better understand an invisible illness that only ensues during pregnancy. Specifically, I address my experiences with the invisible pregnancy-related illness of "incompetent cervix." Through storytelling, I chronicle the illness's definition, impact, diagnosis, subsequent courses of action, and lessons learned. Via candid narration, the chapter's content further illuminates varied perspectives of giving and receiving social support amidst an illness. I begin by describing the lifestage and ensuing events that precipitated the silent illness's discovery.

AN EAGERLY ANTICIPATED LIFESTAGE

Being an African-American woman professor at a majority-race institution is not always easy. The scholarly literature is filled with anecdotal accounts of how this marginalized population is the most overworked, stressed out, underrepresented, and least satisfied of all faculty within university systems (Benjamin, 1997; Bradley, 2005; Gilchrist, 2011a; Malveaux, 1998; Stanley, 2006). On top of these challenges, African-American women professors encounter many dating and mating challenges resulting from work-life balance, negative stereotypes, lack of compatible heterosexual African-American men, identity negotiation, and the Strong Black Woman myth, just to name a few (Gilchrist, 2011b). Pressures of life in the academy compounded by the plethora of dating and mating challenges have led many African-American women professors to delay or even forgo having children (Gilchrist, 2011b). I was a member of this exclusive club for many years, but as I entered my mid-thirties, I decided to prioritize family. Though my career was my first love, I refused to let it be my sole love. After much time, prayer, and internal reflection, I met and soon married my husband. So at the prime of my life, I took inventory: tenure in the professoriate, check; husband, check; house, check; baby, no check. I essentially had all the major things I wanted in life except a baby. As my only salient unchecked desire, motherhood became my prime objective.

Motherhood is commonly viewed as the "pinnacle of womanhood" and a "site of power" for women (O' Reilly, 2004, p. 10). I was a true reflection of these statements and had a fire in my womb that desired to give birth more than anything. My husband had an equal passion for children and embraced fatherhood with an open mind and heart. Extant literature that alleges fathers and mothers in the U.S.A. overall play similar parental roles (e.g., Borisoff, 2005; Douglas & Michaels, 2004; Golden, 2001; Phares, 1999) truly reflected us, as we were tit-for-tat in our parental desires. Because a baby was our only missing piece of the puzzle, my husband and I decided to try immediately for a baby after we married. To our surprise and delight, we conceived during our honeymoon! We were elated, and our elation soon turned to exuberant joy when we found out during our first ultrasound that we were having twins! Months later the gender scan revealed that we would soon be the proud and long-awaited parents of twin girls. We wanted nothing more than to mother and father the precious angels that both of us had waited a lifetime to behold. Though we were older first-time parents, the pregnancy progressed well, and we were well on our way to becoming an actual mom and dad.

I have always had a type-A personality, which is characterized as being very competitive and time urgent (Friedman, 1996). In true type-A personality form, once I learned the babies' genders I began preparing for their arrival. I picked out names, ordered nursery furniture, bought clothes, researched pediatricians, and simply planned a future that included them. As icing on the cake, once I got out of the first trimester, my morning sickness subsided, my energy elevated, and in spite of maintaining a full-time teaching and research load and getting bigger each day, I felt overall good and was loving this particular lifestage. Though their arrival was still a few months away, I wanted to do everything possible to prepare for my sweet girls and ensure their health and safety. I never missed a doctor's appointment, I followed the doctor's orders, took my prenatal vitamins, and looked forward to each ultrasound so that I could check their progress. All signs were positive; I visibly looked like a very healthy mother-to-be, and having made it five-and-a-half months into the pregnancy, all indicators alluded to an approaching normal and healthy dual birth. Little did we know, an invisible illness was brewing inside of me and would soon change our lives forever.

LIFESTAGE INVISIBLE ILLNESS REVEALS ITSELF

It was the eve of Halloween. We had purchased candy in anticipation of trick-or-treaters the following day. I went to work and taught two classes at the university. Given that I was getting bigger and further along in the pregnancy with the twins I was indeed tired but made it through the work day quite well. I went home after work, cooked and ate dinner, spent time with my husband, prepared for the next work day, and went to bed. It was simply my normal daily routine, but what ensued was far from the norm. At almost exactly 5 a.m., I was awakened by a wet sensation. Startled, I jumped out of bed. I cried out to my husband and shouted, "I'm leaking!" "What do you mean?" he asked. "I'm leaking! What's wrong with our babies?" I proclaimed in terror.

Within five minutes we were in the car rushing to the emergency room. I called my parents in route, and they met us at the hospital. By the time I checked in, it was quite evident that my water had broken and I was in preterm labor. I was now confronted with a barrage of paperwork, lab tests, and questions—questions that I could not answer. After all, everything seemed fine leading up to this point. I had no known illnesses, and my lab work, ultrasounds, and monthly checkups had all been essentially perfect. So why was this happening? My family was determined to find out what was going on and to do everything possible to save the babies, so they called in an OBGYN specialist, who gave clear instructions: lay flat on your back, don't move, drink tons of water, and pray for a miracle. At twenty-two weeks, I needed to make it at least two more weeks for the babies to stand a chance at survival. At this point, I did not need to be versed in the teachings of Paul Ricoeur (1988), the French philosopher who studied the essence of human time in Volume 3 of *Time and Narrative,* and noted that *cosmological* time involves linear succession. This was an innate process for me, where I had to hope, wish, and pray for at least fourteen more days of womb-housing my babies. Without a doubt, these would be the longest and most tumultuous days of my life.

Day 1: Fearful

Pure fear characterized the first day. Going into pre-term labor was a fear unlike any I had ever experienced. My water breaking offered segue to the fear I would later encounter with the collage of blood tests, physical examinations, and simply waiting to see what would happen. On day one I also had to inform the administration and my colleagues at the university about my unfortunate situation. Word also quickly spread among my family and friends. Everyone was concerned and showered me with calls, emails, visits, well wishes, and prayers. While I felt blessed that so many people were concerned about the babies' and my well-being, I was also fearful of letting everyone down. These were not just the babies of my husband and me; there were grandparents, aunts, uncles, cousins, friends, church and community members who also loved these children and looked forward to being a part of their lives.

My fear was somewhat calmed by the doctors' swift actions. They were constantly monitoring me and gave me magnesium sulfate, the labor suppressing drug (Viamontes, 1996), in the hope of preventing my uterus from contracting and allowing the babies the precious time needed to develop. With time and increased water intake, amniotic fluid can regenerate (American Pregnancy Association, 2016b). My objective was to gulp down as much water as I could throughout the day and lay flat without even the slightest incline so that that none of the regenerated amniotic fluid would leak out. Stiff from lying down all day the thought of a pillow to elevate my head was refreshing but not permissible. With no signs of contractions and the leaking amniotic fluid seemed to stop finally, some of my fear slowly transitioned to hope, and I became more optimistic that I could endure the difficult journey ahead. Day 1 down, thirteen more to go.

Day 2: Hopeful

The doctors, nurses, my family, and I were all hopeful on the second day that I could carry the babies long enough for them to be placed in the neonatal intensive care unit. The researcher in me wanted to learn as much about my situation as I could. My main question centered on why this happened. No one had answers at the time. I was told we could explore the cause of the problem later, but this critical time needed to be devoted to mitigating the problem. Nonetheless, I could not suppress my inquisitive nature. My family researched pre-term labor on the Internet and reported their findings to me. I also asked the nurses how many successful cases they had encountered. From our research efforts and impromptu inquiries, we found many positive results. Social Comparison Theory (SCT), first proposed by Leon Festinger (1954), alleges individuals determine their social and personal worth by comparing themselves to similar others. In line with the overall premise of SCT, I told myself that if other mothers survived preterm labor to have healthy children ultimately, then I could too. The competitive type-A personality (Friedman, 1996) in me would not have it any other way—no way would I be content with other mothers fighting and succeeding for their unborn babies, while failure plagued me. So not only was I hopeful on Day 2, I was determined. Day 2 down, twelve more to go.

Day 3: Helpless

Shortly after midnight on the third day following the amniotic sac's rupture, things took a turn for the worst. I began to have adverse reactions to the labor suppression drug, (i.e., magnesium sulfate). I was initially prescribed a high dosage of it in an attempt to keep the contractions at bay, but after being on the drug for forty-eight hours, my body began to reject it. Adverse reactions to magnesium sulfate are relatively common and often include sweating, extreme thirst, hypotension, confusion, muscle weakness, and respiratory depression, just to name a few (Viamontes, 1996). I experienced all of the aforementioned side effects, with the most troubling including difficulty regulating my body temperature, causing me to teeter between hot and cold extremities. To mitigate these effects, the dosage of magnesium sulfate was greatly reduced and, in return, my uterus began to contract. With each premature contraction, I knew labor was imminent, yet I refused to let my babies go.

As the day progressed, the labor pains intensified, and the fate of my unborn babies became increasingly bleak. Once the membranes in the amniotic sac have been ruptured for more than twenty-four hours, there is an increased chance of infection (Seward et al., 1998). My rising temperature informed the medical team that my body had become infected, which was later verified by blood work that indicated an elevated white blood count. At this point, the doctors informed my family and me that hope was lost, and we needed to deliver the babies. "No!" I protested. "You cannot take my babies!" My position was momentarily respected, but with each passing hour, I became decreasingly able to speak for myself and my unborn babies.

The combination of medications, contractions, rising infection, and helplessness took a toll, and I began to drift in and out of consciousness. After hours of suffering, the doctors informed my family that if the babies were not soon delivered, there was a chance of losing not only the babies but also losing me. At that point, my husband consented to proceed with delivery. I was coherent just enough to understand that my dream of mothering these sweet innocent girls had been deferred and was drying up like a raisin in the sun[1]. As the medical team prepared me to give birth, I made one final plea. "Please try to save at least one of my babies," I begged out of pure desperation. Surely this was a reasonable request, given that I was having fraternal twins with each in her own sac. The ultrasound revealed that while one baby's sac had punctured, the other was fully intact. So though I had no choice but to accept that I would lose one baby, I desperately prayed the other would survive.

The anesthesiologist gave me an epidural for pain management during the labor and delivery process. I rhetorically asked myself, "These medications will numb my body, but what will numb my heart?" No drug exists for that level of pain. Within what seemed like only a matter of minutes it was time to push. Three pushes and the first baby was out. The nurse placed her lifeless yet warm body in my arms. "I'm so sorry baby; I'm so sorry that I failed you," I apologetically cried out to her 0.9-pound body. In the midst of cradling my baby and apologizing to her, I heard a pop and felt a gush of fluid. The doctor had manually broken the sac that housed my second daughter. "Oh no, they are not even going to try to save the second baby," I cried. "We need you to push again," the doctor said. Just like before, three pushes and the second baby was out, weighing in at just only 1 pound. So there I lay—tired, weak, sick, and holding the breathless bodies of my two beautiful daughters. I was inconsolable; did I just "give birth to death"? (Mondragon, 2012). It felt like this was a twisted nightmare, but the brokenness in my heart, the look on my husband and parents' faces, and the two bodies I held made it clear that this was not a nightmare from which I could awaken. My dream had not only been deferred; it had been nullified.

THE NULL EFFECT

The Communication Research Methods course is the main class I teach. Whenever we study Hypothesis Testing in the course, I explain to my students the *null hypothesis*, which is viewed as a hypothesis of no difference that denies or negates a research hypothesis. Whereas the research hypothesis establishes a relationship or difference among variables, the null hypothesis presumes "no difference" or "no relationship" among the variables (Wimmer and Dominick, 2014). The null hypothesis, in sum, supposes a state of nothingness. Following the miscarriage, I felt like nothing more than a null hypothesis.

In my mind, my womb had been robbed. My babies were supposed to be there still, warm and nestled in protection. Instead, they were placed in a cool freezer so their bodies would not decay while we decided the next steps. My body was zoned out, grieving, and I simply wanted to pull the covers over my head and sleep indefinitely, yet my heart knew I had to be present for my babies and perform some very difficult acts. For example, the nurse asked if we wanted to dress them and take some pictures. Talk about a dialectical tension! Baxter's (1990) dialectical theory alleges there are contradictions in interpersonal relationships. As stated by Lusk (2008), human engagement is characterized by "the interplay of perceived opposite forces or contradictions and . . . communicators [must] negotiate these ever-changing processes" (p. 3). In true dialectical form, we knew it would be extremely painful to hold, dress, and take pictures with our daughters, but we also knew this would be our only opportunity to engage in such precious activities shared between parents and children. So how could we say no? As grief-stricken as we were, we could not deny ourselves these fleeting moments with our babies. Their bodies were lifeless, yet so innocently gorgeous. They were now beginning to change colors, but that didn't matter; they were still our beautiful babies, and we loved them no matter what. For the first and only time, my husband and I dressed them in matching pink dresses and placed tiny bonnets on their heads. The hospital staff also provided tiny cloth bunnies, and we cradled one under each of their arms. My husband and I then huddled close together, and the nurse snapped our only family portrait. After a few more precious moments together, my family thought it would be best for the nurse take them back so we could finalize their arrangements. Never did I want to let them go—I wanted to hold my babies forever, but that was not an option. So amidst what seemed like an endless flow of tears, I kissed and placed them in the nurse's arms.

Once I composed myself, it was time to make some difficult decisions—what to do with their remains. After weighing the available options, we ultimately decided to cremate our daughters and have a small memorial service. I called the funeral home and asked the director to come to the hospital to pick up our daughters and initiate arrangements for their cremation and memorial service. No one told me exactly when the funeral home worker arrived to pick up our daughters, but an even deeper emptiness activated in me around the time they left. It was as though my spirit innately detected an increased physical distance. When the nurse entered my room and informed me that the babies were gone, she again offered her condolences for what we were experiencing and proceeded to say that one of the saddest parts of her job is seeing bad things happen to good people. While I was fighting with everything in me to save our babies, a drug addicted mother was also delivering her baby, according to the nurse. In spite of the mother using drugs throughout her pregnancy, she managed to carry the baby full term. My insides screamed at the mere thought of this injustice, and I was immediately consumed with envy. Envy is marked by desire, where one wants what another person has (Gerrod Parrott and Smith, 1993). I would never dream of drinking, smoking, or doing drugs while pregnant. Instead, I maintained a healthy diet, took my prenatal vitamins, made all of my scheduled doctor's appointments, exercised appropriately, and made a valiant effort to research and apply techniques for ensuring a healthy pregnancy. Yet, in spite of my best efforts, I lost two babies while another mother who was the complete antithesis of health and wellness during pregnancy carried her baby full term. "Where's the justice?" I asked in vain.

As the day evolved, I suppressed some of my envious emotions and began to focus on healing so that I could go home. Within forty-eight hours, the infection subsided, my white blood count normalized, and I was discharged. I couldn't stand being in the same hospital where our babies perished, so I welcomed my release, but a part of me deeply dreaded going home without them. I knew I would struggle seeing their nursery and going through their belongings, but I never imagined exiting the hospital would be so difficult. To exit the maternity ward, I was wheeled down a long corridor filled with pictures of newborn babies. Many of the pictures also featured parents embracing and kissing their new additions. The families looked so happy, and the babies all appeared healthy and vibrant. Again, I was stricken with envy. I wanted our happy family portrait to grace the hospital's corridor, but instead, I was surrounded by images of life and happiness, all while existing in a personal hell. I was simply amazed that with the wealth of knowledge doctors, nurses, and hospital administrators why has no one implemented an alternative hospital exit strategy for bereaved parents. Surely they know that it is unorthodox for parents to outlive their children (Brenner, 2012). My body was weak, and my heart was shattered into a million pieces, so the last thing I needed was a reminder of what we had lost. I simply closed my eyes, dropped my head, and prayed for an expedient exit.

The next few days were pure torture. I had to return home for the first time without our babies, and the air felt cold, distant, and empty. The cremation and memorial service soon ensued. I can write very little about these events because they're all a blur. I felt like a walking zombie, struggling to get through each taxing event. As a woman of faith, I coped by praying endlessly, but research has alleged that while using personal coping strategies, such as prayer and positive thinking, people also benefit from support provided by members of their social networks (Henderson, Gore, Davis, and Condon, 2003). I socially needed help, and I unapologetically sought it out. After the memorial service, I thumbed through the bereavement package we received at the hospital, which contained literature on how to cope with losing a child and a list of local support groups for grieving parents. *Social support* has been defined as assistance that improves the recipient's welfare (Schumaker and Brownell, 1984); "responsiveness to another's needs, and more specifically, as acts that communicate caring; that validate the other's worth, feelings or actions; or that facilitate adaptive coping with problems through the provision of information, assistance, or tangible resources" (Cutrona, 1996, p. 10); and assistance that helps "the recipient seek realistic alternatives to a stressful situation, gain skills, and recognize that help and resources are available from others" (Robbins and Rosenfeld, 2001, p. 279).

Per my insistence, my husband and I attended a monthly parents' bereavement session. I found it comforting knowing we were not alone, and I gained strength from each couple's story of loss. Together we cried, prayed, and truly empathized with each other. While this meeting provided such a source of strength and social support for me, I found the outside world just didn't get it. I cringed whenever people tried to rush me to simply "get over it." I grew to hate the following phrases: "It will get better with time;" "Be strong;" "They are in a better place;" and the worst of all, "I know how you feel." No! You do not know how I feel because everyone feels different when going through difficult life events. Though they had good intentions, many attempts at social support from my family and peer groups failed miserably. The social support that I valued most occurred when people would simply let me talk on my time and terms. I also appreciated when people said, "I can't imagine what you are going through;" "I'm praying for you;" and "You *will be* a great mother soon." These comments came from individuals Parrott (2001) labels *advocates*, who use honest and sensitive comments to bring comfort through a genuine loving presence, and they offer grieving parents practical, hands-on help. The social support I received from these *advocates* little-by-little helped me release myself from this null effect and begin to heal mentally and physically. However, I knew I would never experience authentic healing until the invisible lifestage illness was identified.

LIFESTAGE INVISIBLE ILLNESS IDENTIFIED

Two weeks after the miscarriage, I returned to my OBGYN. She was very apologetic regarding our loss, but these were empty words I did not care to hear. Two good things happened during this visit. First, my physical body seemed to be healing well, with no sign of infections or other visible illnesses. Second, I decided during that appointment to take ownership of my health and do whatever was needed to not let my daughters' loss be in vain. It started by having a respectful, yet candid conversation with my OBGYN. I asked her a simple question, "What caused this?" She responded, "I don't know; it could just be one of those things." I then proceeded to tell her that placentas don't rupture five-and-a-half months into a pregnancy for no reason, and we needed to know what happened before we could ever be comfortable trying for another child. I did everything I was told to do to have a healthy pregnancy, yet this happened. It was clear that she had no answers for me, so I left and never returned to her office.

When I got home, I called the high-risk OBGYN who consulted during the miscarriage. I asked him to please take me on as his patient. He agreed, and I had my first visit a couple of weeks later. During that initial appointment, he asked a collage of questions. I was impressed that he seemed to care this much about my overall health. He also performed many blood tests and scheduled me for an ultrasound. Within days, I received news that all my blood cultures were normal. On the one hand, I was relieved, but I still did not know what illness plagued my pregnancy. A few days later, I went in for my scheduled ultrasound. I was hopeful that I would finally get an answer, but yet I had ultrasounds throughout the pregnancy that revealed no abnormalities. This ultrasound, however, would be different. The doctor and technician meticulously examined me, and after several minutes the doctor looked at me and said the words I needed to hear: "I know why you miscarried. You have an incompetent cervix."

"What's an incompetent cervix?" I asked. I had never heard of that. The doctor informed me that many women are unaware of it because it's not an illness for them unless they become pregnant and have late-term complications carrying the baby. The doctor proceeded to define an incompetent cervix as cervical insufficiency or a weak cervix that contributes to premature birth or pregnancy loss in an otherwise healthy pregnancy (Mayo Clinic, 2015). It affects about 1 to 2 percent of all pregnancies (American Pregnancy Association, 2016a). The doctor further explained that my weakened cervix coupled with the added weight of two babies caused my cervix to dilate prematurely, resulting in early labor. Though this was troubling news to receive, I breathed a sigh of relief—at least my lifestage invisible illness had finally been identified. Now, a plethora of questions flooded my mind, but the question I needed answered most was, "Will I be able to have children, given my incompetent cervix?" The doctor brought some ease to my mind when he informed that many women with an incompetent cervix had delivered healthy babies through the assistance of a *cerclage*, which are strong sutures that enclose and provide support for the weakened cervix (Mayo, 2015). Having clearly identified the invisible illness, as well as a solution, the doctor told us whenever we were ready, we could try again to become pregnant. We were overjoyed to hear these words, yet lingering fear of history repeating itself remained; truly, a journey confronted us.

LIFESTAGE INVISIBLE ILLNESS AND THE 37-AND-ONE-HALF WEEK JOURNEY

Less than two months after getting the green light from the doctor to pursue pregnancy again, we were pregnant. Conception was easy-breezy, but now the hard part ensued—I had to carry the baby to term amidst haunting memories of the past. During the miscarriage, time was not on our side; would time now be our friend or foe? Aside from *cosmological time* (i.e., time moving in linear succession), Ricoeur (1988) alleges there is also *phenomenological time* (i.e., time experienced in terms of the past, present, and future). Ricoeur argues that the two are experienced jointly in that the past, present, and future of phenomenological time presupposes the successive trait of cosmological time. Specifically, the past is always before the present, which is always after the past and before the future. Ricoeur's bifurcation of cosmological and phenomenological time was most fitting to my overall concept of time when I became pregnant again, with the same lifestage invisible illness that resulted in previous heartbreaking results. In other words, the *past* miscarriage of my twin girls at five-and-a-half months into the pregnancy was always before my *present* pregnancy, which was situated after the miscarriage and before the *future*, which we hoped, wished, and prayed would result in a successful pregnancy and birth. This complicated view of phenomenological time became even more convoluted with each thought that my lifestage invisible illness of incompetent cervix was a problem with my past pregnancy, it was an issue with my present pregnancy, and it would always be a concern with any future pregnancies. From the moment I first saw the double lines on the home pregnancy test, I knew it would be the longest and most stressful nine months of my life.

At the first doctor's visit after becoming pregnant again, the doctor marveled at how quickly conception occurred. Then, he told me words I'll never forget: "You've done your part, now let me do my part in helping you get this baby here." Because of my invisible lifestage illness, I was immediately placed in a "high risk" pregnancy category that demanded a plethora of concessions, beginning with surgery to receive the cerclage immediately after the first trimester. Specifically, I received a *McDonald cerclage*, the most common type, involving sutures placed at the upper cervix that are usually removed around the thirty-seventh week of pregnancy (Jazayeri, 2015). I recovered fairly quickly from this procedure and assumed that it was a workable solution for my invisible illness. However, at my next ultrasound a few weeks later, the doctor informed me that he did not think the sutures would suffice for the pregnancy's duration; thus, he wanted to perform another surgical procedure and insert a *Shirodkar cerclage*, which is a lesser performed and more challenging procedure that places more permanent sutures higher up on the cervix that is often not removed prior to delivery, resulting in a cesarean section (1, 2005).

I was highly troubled at the thought of having another surgery. If the first surgery did not mitigate the invisible illness, how could we be sure that this one would? After much research, prayer, and consultation with my social support system, I consented to the second surgery. This surgery taxed me much more than the previous one. While I recovered in a matter of days from the McDonald cerclage, it took weeks to recuperate following the Shirodkar cerclage. Fortunately, follow-up ultrasounds suggested promising news that the cerclage would endure the pregnancy, but carrying a baby to term given my invisible illness would still require many behavior alterations on my part, such as avoiding climbing stairs, long periods of standing, intercourse, and traveling more than an hour. In addition to the things I could not do, there was a litany of things I had to do: daily hip shots of progesterone (i.e., a hormone produced by the ovaries that is essential for supporting the pregnancy and establishing the placenta; Briggs, Freeman, and Yaffe, 2011), have twice-monthly and sometimes weekly doctor's appointments, and receive frequent ultrasounds to monitor the baby's status and my cervix. Mitigating my lifestage invisible illness was arduous and beyond stressful. I question if I could have survived without my social support system, which came in the forms of prayer, encouragement from my immediate family, and face-to-face and virtual communication with other women who had incompetent cervix.

Granted, a normal pregnancy is composed of forty weeks, but given my lifestage invisible illness, the doctor simply wanted to get me to a stage where the baby was fully developed and could bypass the neonatal unit. I had an ultrasound around thirty-six weeks, which indicated the baby was developed enough to proceed with delivery, especially since I had received betamethasone earlier in the pregnancy, which is a steroid that helps the baby's lungs develop (Briggs et al., 2011). So at thirty-seven-and-one-half weeks, I delivered via cesarean section because my cerclage remained throughout the pregnancy. I was overjoyed and blessed to give birth to a healthy six-pound, ten-ounce daughter, who we named London after her deceased sisters (i.e., Landri and Logan)[2] and after the majestic city of London, England. When I held her for the first time I was consumed with gratefulness and relief. It was a desperately long and painful journey, riddled with much uncertainty, but my lifestage invisible illness ultimately did not keep us from reaching our most treasured goal of becoming biological parents. Instead, it empowered me with knowledge that I now embrace and eagerly share with others.

LESSONS LEARNED FROM A LIFESTAGE INVISIBLE ILLNESS

I have learned four crucial lessons from my lifestage invisible illness. First, losing our twin daughters was the most salient mortality experience I have endured. A husband or wife who loses a spouse is labeled a widow; likewise, when a parent dies that child is called an orphan. However, our vernacular is void of a label for parents who lose a child. Perhaps this is the case because "in the natural order of things, parents are not meant to bury their children" (Brenner, 2012, para. 1). Consequences of my lifestage invisible illness taught me a haunting lesson about unnatural mortality, but somehow through my pain and despair, I learned, secondly, to own my health. I quickly learned that I had to be my own advocate; no longer would I assume I was healthy and blindly take the advice of medical professionals. I learned to question and research everything, including diagnoses, medications, and surgical procedures, and if I disagreed with a prognosis, I made it known and fought for my health and health of my unborn child. Furthermore, if I deemed a doctor unsatisfactory, I unapologetically disassociated myself from his/her practice.

In other words, my invisible illness taught me the value of health and wellness.

Along with the lessons learned about unnatural mortality and taking charge of my health, I learned that regardless of my type-A personality (Friedman, 1996), I have little if any control over time. I have no control over the linear succession (i.e., *cosmological time*), for if I did, my twin girls would be here. Similarly, I cannot control *phenomenological time*, which is experienced in terms of the past, present, and future (Ricoeur, 1988). Each day I contend with phenomenological time because a day never goes by that I do not think about and miss our twin daughters (past); each day I try to honor the twins by being the best possible mother to our current daughter (present); and, I know that regardless of how much cosmological time passes, I will forever have a lifestage invisible illness that will impact any pregnancies we may consider (future). Given how my lifestage invisible illness has affected my past, present, and future, I learned a fourth lesson: social support is priceless. Particularly, I now know that seeking assistance during stressful times (Robbins and Rosenfeld, 2001) is not symbolic of weakness; instead, it takes a strong person to admit he/she needs to communicate with similar others who empathize and can, consequently, facilitate adaptive coping (Cutrona, 1996). Because I clearly understand the value of social support, I selectively choose who I communicate with about my lifestage invisible illness; I know that it's okay to cry when I'm sad; and, I know it's even more okay to live each day to its fullness and share my story with others.

REFERENCES

American Pregnancy Association. (2016a). "Incompetent cervix: Weakened cervix." Retrieved from http://americanpregnancy.org/pregnancy-complications/incompetent-cervix/

American Pregnancy Association. (2016b). "Low amniotic fluid levels: Oligohydramnios." Retrieved from http://americanpregnancy.org/pregnancy-complications/oligohydramnios/

Baxter, L. A. (1990). "Dialectical contradictions in relationship development." *Journal of Social and Personal Relationships, 7*(1), 79–88.

Benjamin, L. (1997). *Black women in the academy: Promises and perils*. Gainesville, FL: University Press of Florida.

Borisoff, D. (2005). "Transforming motherhood: 'We've come a long way,' maybe." *Review of Communication, 5*(1), 1–11.

Bradley, C. (2005). "The career experiences of African American women faculty: Implications for counselor education programs." *College Student Journal, 39*, 518–527.

Brenner, A. (2012). "When a child dies: Transition through unimaginable loss." *Psychology Today*. Retrieved from http://www.psychologytoday.com/blog/in-flux/201207/when-child-dies

Briggs, G. G., Freeman, R. K., and Yaffe, S. J. (2011). *Drugs in pregnancy and lactation: A reference guide to fetal and neonatal risk* (9th ed.). Philadelphia, PA: Lippincott Williams & Wilkins.

Cutrona, C. (1996). *Social support in couples*. Thousand Oaks, CA: Sage.

Douglas, S. J., and Michaels, M. W. (2004). *The mommy myth: The idealization of motherhood and how it has undermined women*. New York, NY: Free Press.

Festinger, L. (1954). "A theory of social comparison processes." *Human Relations, 7*, 117–140.

Friedman, M. (1996). *Type A behavior: Its diagnosis and treatment*. New York, NY: Plenum Press (Kluwer Academic Press).
Gerrod Parrott, W. W., and Smith, R. H. (1993). “Distinguishing the experiences of envy and jealousy.” *Journal of Personality and Social Psychology, 64*(6). 906–920.
Gilchrist, E. S. (Ed.). (2011a). *Experiences of single African-American women professors: With this Ph.D., I thee wed.* Lanham, MD: Lexington Books.
Gilchrist, E. S. (2011b). “'One of These Things Is Not Like The Others': African American women professors’ experiences with majority-race students.” In M. N. Niles and N. S. Gordon (Eds.), *Still searching for our mothers' gardens: Experiences of new, tenure track faculty of color at 'majority' institutions* (pp. 213–233). Lanham, MD: University Press of America.
Golden, A. G. (2001). “Modernity and the communicative management of multiple roles: The case of the worker-parent.” *Journal of Family Communication, 1*(4), 233–264.
Henderson, P., Gore, S., Davis, B., and Condon, E. (2003). “African American women coping with breast cancer: A qualitative analysis.” *Oncology Nursing Forum, 30,* 641–700.
Jazayeri, A. (2015). “Cervical cerclage.” *Medscape.* Retrieved from http://emedicine.medscape.com/article/1848163-overview#a3
Lusk, H. M. (2008). “A study of dialectical theory and its relation to interpersonal relationships.” *University of Tennessee Honors Thesis Projects.* http://trace.tennessee.edu/utk_chanhonoproj/1206
Malveaux, J. (1998). “Retaining master jugglers.” *Black Issues in Higher Education, 15*, 40.
Mayo Clinic (2015). “Incompetent cervix.” Retrieved from http://www.mayoclinic.org/diseases-conditions/incompetent-cervix/basics/definition/con-20035375
Mondragon, S. (2012). *I give birth to death.* Retrieved from https://www.englishpen.org/outreach/poem-i-give-birth-to-death-by-sara-mondragon/
O’Reilly, A. (2004). *Toni Morrison and motherhood: A politics of the heart*. New York, NY: State University of New York Press.
Parrott, C. (2001). *Parents' grief: Help and understanding after the death of a baby.* Issaquah, WA: Medic Publishing Co.
Phares, V. (1999). *Poppa psychology: The role of fathers in children's mental well-being.* Westport, CT: Praeger.
Ricoeur, P. (1988). *Time and narrative* (K. Blamey and D. Pellauer, Trans.). Chicago, IL: The University of Chicago Press. (Original work published 1983).
Robbins, J. E., and Rosenfeld, L. B. (2001). “Athletes’ perceptions of social support provided by their head coach, assistant coach, and athletic trainer, pre-injury and during rehabilitation.” *Journal of Sport Behavior, 24*(3), 277–297.
Schumaker, S. A., and Brownell, A. (1984). “Toward a theory of social support: Closing the gaps.” *Journal of Social Issues, 40*(4), 11–36.
Seaward, P. G., Hannah, M. E., Myhr, T. L., Farine, D., Ohlsson, A., Wang, E. E., et al. (1998). “International multicenter term prom study: Evaluation of predictors of neonatal infection in infants born to patients with premature rupture of membranes at term. Premature rupture of the membranes.” *American Journal of Obstetrics and Gynecology, 179*(3 Pt 1), 635–639.
Stanley, C. A. (2006). *Faculty of color: Teaching in predominantly white colleges and universities.* Bolton, MA: Anker Pub.
Viamontes, C. M. (1996). “Pharmacologic intervention in the management of preterm labor: An update.” *The Journal of Perinatal and Neonatal Nursing, 9*(4), 13–30.
Wimmer, R. D., and Dominick, J. R. (2014). *Mass media research: An introduction* (10th ed.). Boston, MA: Wadsworth.

NOTES

1. Quoted from Langston Hughes (1951) *Harlem (“What happens to a dream deferred?”)*
2. This chapter is dedicated to the memory of Landri and Logan—forever in my heart.

Chapter Seven

Reframing Personal and Professional Identity in Connection to "Ability"

Cerise L. Glenn

For the third night in a row, I'm in bed staring at the ceiling trying not to move, desperately trying to fall asleep. Every move sends searing pain through my body. I keep hoping for relief to fall asleep before the next wave hits. If I can just get three good hours, I will have enough to function tomorrow. I finally manage to drift off to sleep. The next thing I know, it's morning. Cranky and in pain, I manage to get out of bed. I brace as I apply the topical medication to the flares on my skin. I pull myself together to make it to campus. Later in the afternoon, I prepare for my lecture. I can feel my skin tearing open under my right arm. I again curse in my mind from the excruciating and long recovery from an ill-advised surgery. I force myself to get through the class without stopping, taking relief in the hope that I visit the Wound Care Center again tomorrow. Maybe I will get some better help to heal…

DISABILITY AND SOCIAL IDENTITY

Forms of disability, like other aspects of social identity, become an integral part of how we see ourselves and our interactions with others. Our sense of ability is central to how we convey our identities to others (see Hecht, 1993; Jackson, Glenn, and Morant Williams, 2012). Like social constructs of race and gender, we are often taught to see the world in binary constructs of difference. Often, we are taught to understand them in oversimplified categories that are mutually exclusive. For instance, the construct of gender operates on a male/female binary. We generally learn what one means by framing it as exclusionary and/or the opposite of the other construct. We are also taught to internalize dominant notions of power, which encourages us to see one aspect of identity as more desirable, normative, and physically apparent (Allen, 2011). For aspects of our lives pertaining to ability, the norm of an able body begins before we are born. In medical practice, it is common for parents to screen for abnormalities and at times, they can make decisions on carrying a baby to term depending on the likelihood of certain disabilities. Although historically, health communication scholarship has focused on more documented, well-known disabilities, a growing number of scholars examine rare, chronic, "hidden" illnesses that are often undetectable by early medicinal tests and interventions and may not appear until adolescence or adulthood (see Allen, 2012; Boss and Couden, 2002; Bury, 2008; Defenbaugh, 2013; Rutter and Kiemle, 2014; Vickers, 1997; Williams, 2016).

This chapter examines learning to integrate living with a rare, incurable chronic illness, hidradenitis suppurativa (HS), into my personal and professional identity as a professor. The nature of rare, chronic illnesses makes them difficult to predict and diagnose. HS is one of the more difficult illnesses to examine because it is an auto-immune disease with a wide variety of physical manifestations. Its cause is unknown and without a cure, the best doctors and patients can do is learn what triggers flare ups, treat the skin that flares, and manage the symptoms. Because of this, it often is misdiagnosed, and doctors largely have not been adequately trained to spot and treat it. In my case, I wasn't "officially" diagnosed until my thirties; however, I have suffered from this off and on since adolescence. I went through a painful and fearful round of tests and prospective diagnoses that included biopsies and tests for rare forms of cancer. I was unofficially diagnosed in my twenties while pursuing my master's degree at student health services but was told to find out more when I get "real" health insurance after finishing school. Since I pursued a doctorate immediately after my masters, that would take years. The systemic issues of HS are quite problematic, including taking medication that is "experimental" without much knowledge of long-term effects, having to fly to another state to see my doctor, and disputes with health insurance about covering the costs of certain medications and "out-of-network" doctor visits. The physical toll is also exhausting and frustrating, often entailing managing unknown side effects and interaction effects of multiple medications and procedures, in addition to the pain of flares.

Although the systemic, medicinal issues are quite perplexing, expensive, and overwhelming, the issues about social identity are equally difficult to manage. As Fennell (2012) explains, our society's construction of illness is to get it "fixed" through surgery or pills or die. The nature of chronically persistent illnesses does not fit this social construction, making it difficult for me to understand, as well as its impact on my life and professional and social relationships. Shifting this notion of my identity has been and continues to be quite difficult. Additionally, it is quite difficult for friends, family, and coworkers to understand given how they see my social and professional identity. The Communication Theory of Identity (CTI), specifically the dialectical tensions of the enacted, personal, and group layers of social identity, will be utilized to frame salient personal and professional experiences. CTI centers the communicative nature of self-identity, as well as the social identities we enact when we interact with others. Because identity is dynamic and cannot be separated from communication, it impacts the formation, maintenance, and modification of identity. Furthermore, it serves as a process for externalizing identity (Glenn and Jackson, 2010; Hecht, 1993; Hecht, Jackson, and Ribeau, 2003; Jackson, Glenn, and Morant Williams, 2012). Since identity formation and communication is complex, it often occurs in dialectical tensions, which Goodall and Goodall (2002) explain as the "interaction of two opposing arguments or forces" (p. 181). CTI has mostly been utilized in the field of intercultural communication; however, these tensions serve as a useful frame for the understudied area of negotiating social identity with a rare, chronic illness.

SOCIAL IDENTITY IN CRISIS: ADAPTING TO CHRONIC ILLNESS

When good friends describe me, they use phrases such as: "You're such a go getter," "You are fun to be around," "Fun sense of humor," and "You're always the overachiever." In my family, one cousin nicknamed me the family "Brainiac." It's a nickname I hate and luckily I'm not called that by her anymore; however, my role as the smart one and a role model still seems to stay with me. In my more immediate family, I serve as the "peacekeeper" and mediator. I keep us connected. When I've interacted with teachers and professors over the years, they have remarked: "You're the dream student." "I love having you in class." "You're always prepared." "You never skip class." As CTI asserts, our sense of identity comes from communication with those around us. My sense of self-emerged when I was younger and has stayed pretty consistent. I understand the way people characterized me and learned that I was going to be successful, stay reliable, and was never the one anyone had to worry about.

I've been fortunate enough to feel a deep sense of interpenetration with the different layers of identity, meaning the different aspects of who I connect well (Hecht, 1993; Hecht, Jackson, and Ribeau, 2003; Jackson, Glenn, & Morant Williams, 2012). The social, professional, and familial layers of "me" cohere and I have a solid, overarching sense of self internally, and that I convey to the world. I love my job as a professor. I give my students and my research my best energy. I think it's my gift to the world. Being an introvert who doesn't enjoy large groups or the "pomp and circumstance" of large celebrations, I don't shine in big settings. My talent lies in the smaller moments. I'm good at working individually with students. I enjoy teaching, but it both energizes and drains me. I shine when I connect to students and help them discover their potential. As an African American woman, along with members of underrepresented groups who want to support "up and coming" members of similar backgrounds, it's especially important to me to share with students that they can conduct undergraduate and graduate research projects. They can be honors students. They can obtain advanced degrees if they want, even if they feel like they don't have the money or social support to do so. I have co-published and presented with students. One such collaboration won an outstanding journal article of the year award, showcasing my ability to mentor graduate students while making a significant contribution to research. It's one of my proudest moments. I still stay in touch with this student even though he graduated years ago. We sometimes reminisce about the extra time we spent on this project, including working over the winter holiday break to meet a January 4 revision deadline. The sacrifice of the time was worth it; this is one of his proudest moments as well.

At times when life feels overwhelming, I reflect upon this award-winning work with this student as a testament to what I can do. It then hits me as my HS has grown increasingly severe—I'm not this person anymore. I'm no longer the overachiever who can put in all the extra hours and keep going. The thought crushes me and tears well in my eyes as it starts to sink in. I now have to live with the effects of a failed surgery that was supposed to help "fix" me. I have no energy, and I'm in constant pain. I no longer have the luxury of over-producing. I can barely make it through the day. In fact, sometimes I can't. I'm forced to divide my days into smaller chunks of time to rest and take naps like a five-year old kid. Even with that, I spend my weekends trying to balance catching up on work and recuperating. Since chronic illnesses like HS, can occur in "waves," people with chronic illnesses often appear "normal" on the outside and may try to hide or disguise their flares to mimic normalcy (Defenbaugh, 2013; Williams and Jackson, 2013). Because I adopted this strategy early on, and still do at times, it made it difficult for friends, family, and colleagues to understand the effects of living with a chronic illness. If the people I mentioned above were asked to describe me in the early years of adapting to HS, I feel they'd say things like: Remember when she used to go out with us all the time? Remember how much fun you used to be? We miss seeing you around. Haven't heard from you in a while. It must be the pressure of the job." Most of my close friends (other than those who attended my doctoral program with me) and family don't really understand the notion of a "tenure-clock" or the anxiety that comes with earning promotion and tenure. With great hurt, I realize they assume the job matters more to me than they do. Some relationships fall apart. I feel like I'm falling apart.

As I've had the chance to reflect on this difficult experience, I've come to realize that what affected my life and the perceptions of me from the people in my aforementioned social circles was more than difficulty integrating my chronic illness into my sense of self; it was a failure to manage a glaring identity gap, a conflict of the various layers of social identity (Hecht, 1993; Hecht, Jackson, and Ribeau, 2003; Jackson, Glenn, and Morant Williams, 2012; Jung and Hecht, 2004). I didn't know how to tell people what was happening to me, partly because I had such a difficult time making sense of it myself. Although I chose to suffer in silence, a common occurrence with those suffering from a chronic illness that can be kept "hidden," I slowly concluded that I had to find a way to reclaim and redefine my sense of self as I learned how to live with an incurable autoimmune disease. The following two narratives detail my efforts to break this silence during the long healing process from my surgery and subsequent procedures. They overview the failures of self-silencing, with an effort to find a new voice and re-craft my social identity in the process. This was a long, slow process that took years for me to resolve (and I keep having to work at it), so I chose salient moments from my personal and professional life that reflect the challenges and later success of reframing my social identity as a friend, family member, and professional. They reflect my struggle with the following questions:

1. How do I integrate being chronically ill into my sense of self?
2. How do I (and should I) communicate my changing sense of ability to my family and friends?
3. How can I manage my professional identity and career goals when I've been working at such an incredibly fast pace in my first two years in my job?

As a self-described overachiever, will I look like I failed to live up to my potential as I undergo my reappointment review and move through the promotion and tenure process?

NARRATIVE 1: COMMUNICATING MY CHRONIC ILLNESS TO FAMILY

Learning to find my voice and share my chronic illness was incredibly difficult at first. It still is. I decided to first share my diagnosis outside of my most immediate family with one of my cousins, Shanae, who works in the health care industry. We used to be closer when I was in college and right after I graduated, but we hadn't been in touch as much when I was in graduate school working on my masters and doctoral degrees. After relocating back to North Carolina, we'd connected again. I attended one of her son's events near me. We caught up over dinner and drinks. She told me about a difficult family situation that she'd been going through the past few months. She'd be the perfect person to understand. I'd been supportive of her, so it was time to re-create that into a two-way street. As Williams (2016) describes, social support from close family members can be a vital aspect of learning how to live with a rare, chronic illness. As someone who has worked to be supportive of my family, I was hopeful that I could now utilize their support to mitigate the tensions I was feeling due to growing gap in identity of my past and current self. Given her profession in health care, I believed Shanae would offer a sympathetic ear. When we met for dinner, I decided to tell her at the restaurant. It was time to stop suffering in silence.

> Me: So I've been having some serious health issues. It turns out it's something called hidradenitis suppurativa.

> Shanae: Never heard of it.

I tried explaining it. The pain. The flare ups. I began to stumble over my words as I realized she wasn't getting what I was trying to convey. She sighs and leans back in the booth.

> S: Who isn't in pain sometimes? Back, knees, something or other. We all gotta navigate something.

I felt dismissed but desperately needed my family to understand. My hope was that their understanding of my chronic illness would provide support and encouragement to navigate my shifting identity. We met again a couple of months later at my brother's house. I thought I'd try again. My brother and I are close, and he's been my main familial support. It would be easier to convey what I'm going through when he's there. Clearly something was wrong with the way I tried to express myself and explain the HS. My cousin would get it—I just needed to do a better job of explaining it to her. My attempts at what Defenbaugh (2013) describes as the direct approach did not work with my cousin, so this second attempt reflects the medical approach, which I hoped would be more effective. I had a medical brochure that provided an overview of HS that was phrased much better than what I'd tried to explain last time I saw her in person. I explain that due to the rare illness and lack of awareness in the medical community, few doctors can diagnose and treat HS. I found three specialists in the nation who are leaders in "experimental" treatments and surgical procedures. After extensive research and phone calls, I decided to contact a leading specialist in the field. I handed the brochure to her. I told her how excited I was to see the new doctor and that I'm hopeful that he's taking new patients. I have to travel to Ohio to see him, but hopefully, it would be worth it.

Shanae briefly glanced at it. Barely even glanced at it. She handed it back to me without much comment. Surprised, it finally hit me. She'd never get it. It wasn't just because I was having a hard time finding the words. She didn't want to get it. Our relationship only worked when she wanted me to listen to her when she needed a shoulder for support. She wasn't engaged when I needed the support. I felt hurt and dismissed. If I'm not the strong one helping with her problems, did I even matter to her? I wasn't asking for much--just some understanding and support. How many of my other relationships were like this? How many were this one sided? I obviously needed to make a major shift here. Over the next few months, I tried reaching out to her to explain the HS. After many unreturned calls, I finally got it. I made the point to return her calls when she needed someone to talk to, but the same wasn't the case for how she saw me. Occasionally, I'd get a few "Sorry. I've been busy" texts. When she wanted to talk about her issues, I didn't return her calls either. I just couldn't participate in this relationship anymore this way.

This process of engagement (and disengagement) with my cousin angered, disappointed, and hurt me. As I've processed this situation with more distance and perspective, I realize that my HS was difficult for her to manage because it directly contradicted how she's understood my social identity over the course of our lives. As Williams (forthcoming) asserts, family members can have a difficult time adjusting to a chronic illness as well. Although CTI discusses identity gaps as a construct that is negotiated intrapersonally (Hecht, 1993; Hecht, Jackson, and Ribeau, 2003), my interaction with Shanae illustrates that identity gaps can form interpersonally as well. Our failure to successfully navigate this tension resulted in the termination of our friendship and left us as more distant cousins. As my sense of identity shifts, that does not mean that others will adjust their perceptions of me. Her perception of me and our relationship remained static while I was working to integrate the changes due to my illness into not only my own sense of self but into my personal relationships as well.

When more than a year passed and the holiday season came upon us, she reached out again. Always a sucker for connection at the holiday season, I agreed to meet her for dinner. My brother (who has always been very close and supportive of me) refused to see her and told me not to invite her to his house (where I was staying over the holidays). He didn't understand why I bothered with her anymore. I didn't either, but I felt it wouldn't kill me to have a quick meal with her. When I met her at the restaurant, the first thing she said surprised me:

Shanae: I'm sorry.

Me: About what?

S: Not understanding your HS. My friend has it. It's awful. She had to drop out of school and can barely lift her arms. She's always in pain.

For a minute, I just sat there. It's not that I didn't appreciate the apology. It just didn't seem to right the situation after the past year. I told her about what I'd been through multiple times. She just wouldn't listen.

I asked her why she dismissed it when I was going through it, but now that she knew someone else going through it, she could understand. She shrugged and said it just took her friend's situation to get it. She then launched right back into her personal problems. Nothing had changed. In her mind, I'm still the strong, responsible one who could be her shoulder. She apologized to make herself feel better, not to try to be a better family member to me. As she droned on about her personal life, I knew our relationship was pretty much done. I ask her how she's doing via text from time to time, but I don't give her much time or much of my energy. As I've worked on the recrafting of my sense of self, I was beginning to learn how to take better care of myself by not engaging these situations anymore. Unfortunately, she couldn't change the way she saw me and how our relationship was defined in her eyes. She didn't see *me*. She only saw the *old me* she still wanted me to be. As hard as it was, I let this relationship go. We still see each other from time to time at family events, and we remain friendly, but we're not close. Even though identity negotiation is a dynamic process, it may not be for both parties involved in a relationship. In our instance, Shanae could not adapt to my changing sense of self. I couldn't return to my old sense of self given my health situation.

NARRATIVE 2: RECRAFTING MY PROFESSIONAL IDENTITY

Not only did adapting to HS cause issues in renegotiating my personal identity, but it also significantly impacted my professional identity as a professor. This job entails teaching, conducting research, and various service activities, such as committees. Although this narrative is an autoethnographic narrative regarding my career as a professor, the self-reflexive and critical nature of the analysis (Anderson, 2006) speaks to the professional experiences of other underrepresented groups in professions that are have high amounts of autonomy and are goal-oriented more so than being bound by a time clock, and earn and track hourly sick leave. Part of occupations such as these entails the "price of ambition," which at times comes with high amounts of stress and pressure to achieve success at the expense of longevity (Judge and Kammeyer-Mueller, 2012). Judge and Kammeyer-Mueller (2012) also discuss how variables, such as extroversion and gender, impact ambition as they posit men are more ambitious than women and extroversion is more positively correlated to ambition. As an introverted woman of color, I continue to struggle with how to adjust to the unpredictability and pain of a chronic illness, as well as how this affects others' perception of my shifting notions of self-identity. Pushing through the pain was wearing me down, and I couldn't do it anymore. I had to give my body a break. I learned to reduce certain activities and work through the depression that came with this adjustment. Letting go of the person I was felt extremely difficult. I felt like a failure. I was letting people down.

One of my mentors, a full professor, met with me over coffee at a conference to ask how I'm doing. I had told her about my diagnosis. She's one of the people that pushes me hard to research and publish. After the reaction from some of my family members, such as Shanae, I was unsure of how she would treat me now. I decide not to put on my "tough, brave" face and honestly tell her how I feel and what I've been experiencing with HS. I tell her, "I'm feeling better, but I feel like I'm only 65–70 percent of the person I used to be." She asks me what I mean. I tell her I used to be able to write for twelve-hour blocks at a time. I could write until the wee hours of the morning. I cranked out drafts of papers in a day once I pulled my notes, data, and thoughts together. I could binge write and analyze for two to three days and get completely lost in that world. I would stay to myself and be completely immersed in my work. I can't do that now. On a good day, I can sit for two to three hours without pain creeping in. It starts as a tingling sensation. If I ignore it, it starts to crawl over my body and turn into severe pain. I used to hit my research wall around hour four, but I could push through it and keep going. I don't have that kind of push anymore. I can't even sit for that long anymore. I put myself on such a fast-paced trajectory. What if I can't keep up with it anymore?

Nodding sympathetically, she understands and says, "You have to remember that your 65 percent is better than most people's 100 percent." Now, I'm sure she was saying that partly to make me feel better, but it did help me keep in mind that the notion of "overachiever" has been ingrained in me since a was a child. My parents often told me that as an African American, I had to learn to go above and beyond expectations to be seen as an equal. As a woman of color, learning how to navigate gendered and racial perceptions of my professional identity influences how others in the organization perceive me. This entails notions that I should be more nurturing and caring when interacting with others (see Collins, 2000; Glenn, 2012). My notion of 65 percent is probably what normal people equate to 100 percent given how I learned to situate myself in academic and other professional settings. This opened my eyes to help me realize that life with a chronic illness was going to take some major mental recalibration or I'd burn out in misery.

My mentor also asked me about my personal life. This also helped realize I needed to focus on that, including developing better self-care to balance my personal and professional life. Part of internalizing the notion of being a strong overachiever not only caused me to readjust what this meant to me and how I communicated it to others, but it also made me realize I needed to make some drastic shifts in my professional relationships with others. Like many feminists, I believe in the saying "empowered women empower women (and others)," which is highly integrated into my sense of professional identity. Women and men who believe in mentoring others can often find themselves putting high amounts of energy into developing others (Glenn, 2012). Incorporating better self-care into my daily work life is imperative to mitigating the effects of highly ambitious career plans, such as burn-out and additional health issues (Scott, in press). Some colleagues and students drained all of my energy, which I allowed to happen as it meshed with my long-term notion of self. I found myself putting too much energy into the wrong types of activities and relationships, including students, friends, and family members. I had to reduce the amount of energy I spent with graduate students and colleagues who wanted me to "collaborate," but really wanted me to carry the burden of the work. This was especially difficult with a colleague who was once a very close friend. I had to reduce the number of students I mentored. My mentor wisely advised, "Don't mentor students who don't listen. They don't have to do what you say, but they need to listen to you." Her advice helped me figure out how to remain actively involved in professional activities in a way that still allows for the connection and interpenetration of multiple social identities (Hecht, 1993; Jackson, Glenn, and Morant Williams, 2012).

My mentor's comments also helped me realize I wasn't giving enough restorative time to myself or to the students, friends, and family member who really did support *me* and not the "overachiever" notion. To some—I *wasn't* a good friend or loved one. This was a harsh reality to absorb as I realized I needed to overhaul more than just my work habits. The problem was also part of me and how I see myself. Of course, this is interrelated. My intrapersonal layer of self-definition caused me to enact my identity a certain way (Hecht, 1993; Jackson, Glenn, and Morant Williams, 2012) as they are all interrelated and connected, adjusting one impacts the others and causes me to redefine how I see myself, enact it with others, or choose not to engage certain people or situations.

RECRAFTING MY SENSE OF SELF: NAVIGATING THE BACKLASH AND BENEFITS

Learning how to recraft my identity with a chronic illness has been incredibly challenging, but it has also provided me opportunities to grow as a person and make me more grateful for aspects of my life I once took for granted. I'm still learning how to mitigate the dissonance I experience when I compare my current self to my "old" self. I still work to negotiate the newer identity gaps between these two selves. Learning from the relationship with my cousin has made me more mindful of how I treat my other family members, friends, and colleagues. Although we are not close anymore, I have built closer relationships to two of my other cousins. I am much more understanding of constraints on their time and other issues they navigate in their daily lives. I make sure to take breaks from the grind to call and check to see how people are doing. I also am much better at acknowledging smaller *and* bigger accomplishments. I make time to write the thank you notes and spend time with family and friends that I once considered "lost time" that just happens in the end-of-semester holiday season stress. Just as importantly I've learned to give myself breaks and take joy in the smaller moments in life in addition to accolades and achievements. I engage in more self-care and no longer pull all-nighters to binge write and try to get at least six hours of sleep at night (I still miss binge writing from time to time for some reason).

As a critical scholar, it's helped me own my class privilege that my income and educational, cultural capital allow me to have, which could be an essay on its own. As I've met a few others who have HS, I'm grateful for the ability to see my specialist in Ohio two to three times a year--a one to two-day trip that costs between $500 and $1000 per visit. I have an even deeper sense of empathy for those with health conditions that do not allow them to work full time and have health insurance. I'm grateful for a job that allows me flexibility while maintaining autonomy in my career. For instance, I can teach in the summer if I need to earn money to visit my specialist and medical procedures. I can also take time in the summer to recover from medical procedures when needed. The ability to work from home, such as through teaching online, has given me more options with my time. I can work ten to twelve hours on a "good" day and take a shorter day the next if needed. Since mornings can be rough, I have the option to teach late morning, afternoon, and during the evening. I remain grateful for a career that allows me to mitigate some of the more challenging aspects of shifting my social identity.

There has also been some backlash to recrafting my identity living with a chronic illness. Students and colleagues have had to adjust to me limiting my time working, which means not checking work email on most weekends. I have also removed my work email from my mobile phone, so I don't check it as often. This has come with complaints of me not being as much as a "go getter" as I once was and no longer being a "team player" willing to go the extra mile to help. I've had to let go of some longtime friends who I no longer let drain me of all of my energy. I "look selfish" when I've stopped giving and loaning money, opting to create savings for myself instead in case there is ever a time I need to take leave without pay. Although I still wish I was as strong a "go getter" at times, I remind myself that these changes have allowed me to make positive shifts in self-care that will help promote more longevity in my career and more balanced personal life (Scott, in press).

As years have gone by since my official diagnosis and I've been fortunate enough to be treated by a renowned specialist, I am no longer fearful of the loss of "old" me regarding how it will impact my career and personal relationships. I am still productive, but not in the same way and can work toward interpenetration of my professional and personal identity again (see Hecht, 1993; Jackson, Glenn, and Morant Williams, 2012). Thankfully, I am still able to create fulfilling and award-winning work and have found a new world of opportunities personally and professionally. I have earned promotion and tenure and am learning the ropes of a new administrative role. I have built closer relationships with different family members and friends. I am grateful for new friends, even though it makes me sad at times to think about relationships that no longer exist. I am no longer an advanced, stage 3 as I was in my opening narrative. Although I still have to take medication and may have more procedures and surgery in the future, thankfully, I have been able to slowly increase physical activity (which also helps mitigate stress). I am in much better place and feel well rounded. I still have to navigate flare ups (although less severe and frequently), some fear of unknown long term effects of my medication, and misunderstandings of my illness, I am on a more positive path to successfully integrating this chronic illness into my sense of self.

REFERENCES

Allen, B.J. (2011). *Difference matters*. Long Grove, IL: Waveland Press.

Anderson, L. (2006). "Analytic autoethnography. *Journal of Contemporary Ethnography*, 35(4), 373-395. DOI: 10.1177/0891241605280449

Boss, P. and Couden, B.A. (2002). "Ambiguous loss from chronic physical illness: Clinical interventions with individuals, couples, and families." *Journal of Clinical Psychology*, 58(11), 1351–60.

Bury, M. (2008). "Chronic illness as biography disruption." *Sociology of Health and Illness*, 4(2), 167–182. DOI: 10.111/1467–9566.ep11339939.

Collins, P.H. (2000). Black feminist thought: Knowledge, consciousness, and the poltics of empowerment. New York, NY: Routledge.

Defenbaugh, N.L. (2013). "Revealing and concealing ill identity: A performance narrative of IBD disclosure." *Health Communication*, 58: 159–169. DOI: 10.1080/ 10410236.2012.666712

Fennell, P.A. (2012). *The chronic illness workbook: Strategies and solutions for taking back your life.* Delmar, NY: Albany Health Management Publishing.

Glenn, C.L. (2012). "Stepping in and stepping out: Examining the way anticipatory career socialization impacts identity negotiation of African-American women in academia." In G. Chang, C. G. Gonzalez, Y. Flores-Niemann, A. Harris, & G. Gutierrez y Muhs (Eds.) *Presumed incompetent: The intersections of race and class for women in academia*, (pp.133–141). Boulder, CO: University Press of Colorado.

Glenn, C.L. and Jackson, II, R.L. (2010). "Re-negotiating identity in the field of communication." In S. Allan (Ed.), *Rethinking communication: Keywords in communication research*

(International Communication Association Theme Book Series), (pp. 137–149). Cresskill, NJ: Hampton Press.

Goodall, H.L. and Goodall, S. (2002). *Communicating in professional contexts: Skills, ethics, and technologies*. Belmont, CA: Wadsworth/Thomson Learning.

Hecht, M.L. (1993). "A research odyssey: Towards the development of a communication theory of identity." *Communication Monographs* 60: 76–82.

Hecht, M. L., Jackson, R. L., II, and Ribeau, S. A. (2003). "African American communication: Exploring identity and culture." Mahwah, NJ: Lawrence Erlbaum.

Jackson II, R.L., Glenn, C.L., and Morant Williams, K. (2012). "Self-identity and culture." In A. Kurylo (Ed.), *Inter/Cultural communication: Representation and construction of culture*, (pp. 117–140). Thousand Oaks, CA: Sage Publications, Inc.

Judge, T. A., and Kammeyer-Mueller, J. D. (2012). "On the value of aiming high: The causes and consequences of ambition." *Journal of Applied Psychology*, *97*(4), 758–775. DOI: 10.1037/a0028084.

Jung, E. and Hecht, M. L. (2004). "Elaborating the communication theory of identity; Identity gaps and communication outcomes. *Communication Quarterly*, 52(3), 265–283.

Rutter, S.J. and Kiemle, G. (2004). "Exploring the social and interpersonal experience of South Asian women with a diagnosis of systematic lupus erythematosus." *Psychology & Health*, 30(3), 318–335. DOI: 10.1080/08870446.2014.972397.

Scott, K. (in press). *The language of strong Black womanhood: Myths, models, messages and a new mandate for self-care*. Lexington.

Vickers, M.H. (1997). "Life at work with 'invisible' chronic illness (ICI): The 'unseen,' unspoken, unrecognized dilemma of disclosure." *Journal of Workplace Learning*, 9(7), 240–252.

Williams, K. M. and Jackson, R. L. (2013). "The Big Bad Wolf: Lupus, Identity & African American Women." In J. Conyers (Ed.), *Race, Gender, and Identity* (pp. 65–80). Piscataway Township, NJ: Transaction.

Williams, K. M. (2016). "My sister's keeper: Sibling social support and chronic illness. *Journal of Medical Humanities*. DOI: 10.1007/s10912–016–9394–4

Williams, K.M. (forthcoming). "But you look fine: The impact of family social support on African American women living with lupus." *Howard Journal of Communications*, (TBA).

Chapter Eight

Duty, Honor, Country...Sickness

Finding Strength in My Personal Battle with Gulf War Illness

Elizabeth Desnoyers-Colas

In 1962, when Five Star US Army General Douglas MacArthur intoned the three words "duty, honor, country" in his historic speech to West Point cadets he invoked the ultimate sacrificial creed all military officers then and today pattern their careers and lives after. Elaborating on the significance of the phrase he explained, "Those three hallowed words reverently dictate what you ought to be, what you can be, what you will be. ...They build your basic character" (MacArthur, 1962, para. 4).

As a third generation military service person and US Air Force (USAF) officer for almost sixteen years, I was no exception; I solemnly took this creed and stoically applied it to all of my associated duties and missions through my entire Air Force career. It was not easy. Few outside of the military knows that this type of single-minded sacrifice sometimes comes with a heavy cost. Looking back, my stalwart following of General Douglas's unyielding mantra encouraging dedicated military service to this nation, ultimately cost me my health.

I was not alone, however. Hundreds of service members returned to the United States after Operations Desert Shield/ Desert Storm in the early 1990s experiencing a host of unexplained illnesses and debilitating health problems. The media initially dubbed this medical phenomenon the "Gulf War Syndrome," later calling it "Gulf War Illness (GWI)." These associated illnesses included individual symptoms such as headaches, memory loss and cognitive difficulties, skin lesions, rashes, fatigue, muscle and joint pain, and gastrointestinal disorders. Those service members suffering from GWI also had such chronic multi-symptom illnesses as fibromyalgia (FMS), chronic fatigue syndrome (CFS), and multiple chemical sensitivity (MCS). In 2010, the Congressional Committee on Gulf War and Health christened the cluster of maladies as Chronic Multi-Symptom Illness (CMI). The new official name signified both the government's and medical communities' inability to determine the origin of these numerous illnesses and the difficulty with treating them. Although the Department of Veteran Affairs continues to refer to the maladies as CMI, most veterans who suffer from these illnesses today still prefer using the term Gulf War Illness. Today, one in four veterans of the Operation Desert Shield/Desert Storm conflict who served in the Southwest Asia Theater has GWI or CMI (*Report Brief*, Institute of Medicine of the National Academies, January 2013, pp. 1–4). I am one of them.

This autoethnographic personal narrative account outlines the elements of my twenty-five-year journey as an African American female USAF officer who served in Saudi Arabia during Operation Desert Storm and contracted Gulf War Illness, a seemingly invisible illness.

METHOD

Everyone has spoken for the black woman, making it difficult to speak for themselves (Collins, 2000). Yet, African American women are no strangers to storytelling or sharing their own personal narratives. Historically, African American women icons have strongly advocated crafting, sharing, and preserving their own narratives. In her 1892 book, *A Voice from the South*, African American feminist and historian Anna Julia Cooper told African American women that they needed to gather their history and muster the creativity and ingenuity to develop and cultivate their own collective literary and rhetorical voice. Cooper's fundamental fear was that black women's individual and collective life stories and experiences would be ignored and dismissed by white men and women, as well as, by African American men. Almost a century later, black feminist bell hooks (1989) echoes Cooper's admonition, also urging African American women to speak up and out about themselves and significant facets of their lives. Doing so, hooks suggests, would prevent having African American women's histories and life experiences deemed insignificant or rendered invisible. Cultivating and framing the overall constructs of these personal narratives and stories gives black women their own voice, a unique identity and bolsters their ability to tell and legitimize their own to a multitude of audiences.

Stern (2015) notes that personal narratives are a fundamental part of feminist research that can help bring individual and collective marginalized voices to the forefront. Personal narratives, according to Spieldenner (2014) and Hudson (2015) also help to combine an authoethnographer's self within a cultural context. This cultural context can then be used to examine an intersectional identity such as a black woman's multidimensional identity as a military officer serving during Desert Storm, in Saudi Arabia, who contracted GWI.

Autoethnography scholars believe that personal narratives are extremely personal and can be viewed as imperfect. Sparkes (2000) suggests that "auto-ethnographies are highly personal accounts that draw upon the experience of the author researcher for the purposes of extending sociological understanding…taking the question of voice and representation a step further we could argue that an individual is best suited to describe his or her own experience more accurately than anyone else" (p. 21). Personal narratives told by military women from all races and backgrounds, serving in combat zones are unique since women did not typically serve in these roles in great numbers until the 1990s. Consequently, a personal narrative told by an African American female U S Air Force officer who served in a combat zone during Operation Desert Storm in Saudi Arabia and contracted Gulf War Illness is even more unique. This uniqueness is related to the paucity of black female officers who might be willing or even able to share such personal narratives about such causalities of war. The distinctiveness of such stories cannot be discounted. Rose (1994), suggests personal narratives and stories about African American women are important because "it is crucial to have access to more stories by black women, told in such a way that they not only illuminate the lives and social forces that shape them but also allow a given story's messy seams to show, let the many life threads that run through them remain visible. (p. 9)"

SICKNESS AS SACRIFICE: DENYING, BATTLING GWI/CMI

In the summer of 1991, I was at the peak of my military career. I had been notified that I would be promoted to Major, I would become a field grade officer sometime within 1992. As an African American female, I was especially proud of this achievement primarily because I was the first woman military officer in my family. As an African American woman, I knew that making Major would not be an easy task. In those eleven years, I had gone from being the only woman cadet and one of two African American cadets in my forty-person AFROTC detachment at Central Washington University, Ellensburg Washington. I moved on to become the only African American female leader at Eaker Air Force Base, Blytheville, Arkansas who reported directly to the 97th Bombardment (97BMW) Wing Commander.

As a senior USAF captain and third generation military, many African American service women were foundational legacies as I advanced in my military career. During World War II, the African American Press and Civil rights activist Dr. Mary McLeod Bethune was instrumental in waging a relentless hands-on campaign to get African American women to serve in all the services. National politicians knew Bethune, president and founder of the National Council of Negro Women, as an advocate for minorities and the oppressed. The presidential administrations of Coolidge and Hoover had appointed her to government positions. She was especially close to Franklin Roosevelt and his wife, Eleanor and became President Roosevelt's special advisor on minority affairs. With Mrs. Roosevelt's assistance, Bethune successfully used this position as a powerful political platform to persuade the president to allow black women to serve in the military. A very restrictive military service quota (10 percent of the African American population at the time) meant that very few would serve. The Women's Army Auxiliary Corps was founded in 1942; it was quickly renamed the Women's Army Corps in 1943. That year, forty African American women, dubbed the "ten percenters," went to Fort Des Moines, Iowa, for their initial officer training. As part of Dr. Bethune's strategic plan to propel African American women into military service leadership, she and other prominent black leaders carefully handpicked and screened the applicants. Failure was not an option for the African American women of the first female officer candidate class (Desnoyers-Colas, 2014). These women and the others who later joined them in Fort Des Moines over the next three years were constantly watched, evaluated, and probed for any physical, mental, or moral weakness that would discredit their race. In 1942, Charity Adams became the first black WAAC commissioned officer. Over the next three years at Fort Des Moines, Adams built a national reputation as an expert supervisor, trainer, and commander of African American servicewomen (Desnoyers-Colas, 2014). I had been a second lieutenant at my first duty station, Nellis AFB, Las Vegas Nevada, living in the service shadow of Charity Adams for about six months when I was summoned to the new squadron commander's, (an African American female senior captain destined to retire eventually as a Colonel) office.

My meeting with her was anything but a "warm sistah to sistah" encounter. When I walked into her office and saluted, she did not invite me to sit after she returned the salute. She sat and eyed me coolly looking me up and down with barely disguised disdain, as I stood at attention in front of her desk rigid with fear. For the next thirty minutes, still standing at attention, she told me that I had become an "embarrassment" to the other African American officer and enlisted women on this very large base because I was wearing what I jokingly up until then, called a "half fro." She told me that if I wanted to have a successful career in my field, I had to realize that I was highly visible in this position and working for those who worked directly for the two-star General that commanded the base. "The general knows where all of the raisins are in his tapioca pudding," she said gravely. Noting the puzzled look on my face, she further explained that as a black woman working in a field where I would have to speak well, write well, and exude maximum confidence and poise in the presence of senior government officials, international leaders, and community members. Therefore, my hair would have to conform to military regulations. My uniforms and the way that I wear them must be pristine. Like all the black women who had served before us, she said, I would have to know and accept that I would always be watched and judged. "Black service women don't just represent themselves; good or bad, well or sick, they represent "the race," she said with emphasis. If I couldn't handle it, she warned, she would help me leave the Air Force and open the door for another young black woman who could. Ignoring the welling tears in my eyes, she curtly dismissed me, and I saluted her. Under all the *spit and polish* tough demeanor she exhibited, I eventually found out she did have a heart and was concerned. Instead of receiving what could have been a career ending letter of reprimand, she talked my boss into making my time with her (ordered at his behest) a counseling session. Chastened, I got my very nappy, borderline unkempt "half fro" cut and permed into an acceptable military regulation hairstyle for career black women the next day. Lieutenant Colonel Charity Adams would have been proud.

With my hair neatly permed in August 1991, I volunteered to go to Riyadh, Saudi Arabia to serve in the ongoing Gulf War. Many of the people from my base had already gone to combat, and I wanted to go as well. This was the war where American military women, en masse would be able to serve for the first time in combat zones. Ultimately, forty thousand women were sent overseas in direct support of Operations Desert Shield and Desert Storm. Forty percent of them were African American females (Desnoyers-Colas, 2104). I never made it to Riyadh. Before I arrived in Saudi Arabia, I found out that I had been quickly transferred to the U S Central Command Air Forces (CENTAF Forward) Headquarters in Dhahran, Saudi Arabia, because of "cultural and gender sensitivities." Apparently, before I had even left the U S, Brigadier General Eugene D. Santarelli, (who was to be my boss during my time in the desert), had decided that my being female would ultimately hinder my working effectiveness in Riyadh as an Air Force public affairs/protocol officer. Working in the Saudi Arabian capital, I would encounter very senior male members of the Royal family and the all-male ultra-conservative mutaween, (the Saudi Arabian government appointed religious police) who did not like working in any fashion with women, especially foreign ones. While in Riyadh I would not be allowed to drive, and I would not be allowed to speak directly to Saudi military senior officers on behalf of the military. I would have to wear the abaya, (a floor length black gown covering) and a hijab (a scarf to put around my neck and cover my hair) over my military uniform in their presence. I would have to always be accompanied by a US male military escort of any rank who would have to do all the talking for me. In Dhahran, however, military women could drive and did not have to wear abayas. The military climate there for women was more relaxed because of the Western presence of US oil companies, and also most of the Saudi military male officers there had gone to US and British schools and were used to dealing with women in leadership roles. In fact, the only concession made to the mutaween in Dhahran was that US servicewomen and other coalition force females had to wear their military headgear when they drove any military vehicles. Officer and enlisted women also needed to have a male escort with them when conducting face-to-face business with a Saudi male. Ultimately, I came to see the wisdom of General Santarelli's decision to bring me to Dhahran. For me, it would prove to be a win-win job position, higher than the one I would have taken in Riyadh. I did not want to be sent home because I was a woman and this switch allowed me to complete the mission.

I had only been at CENTAF for a few weeks when an Air Force fighter jet assigned to the 4404th (Provisional) Wing crashed while enforcing the No-Fly Zone. The pilot safely ejected from the plane. A routine military aircraft crash board investigation determined that a plane component had malfunctioned. I worked with a representative of the US Central Command Public Affairs (USCENTCOM) Air Force department representative (to gather and dispense approved information for national and international media) to dispel quickly rumors that the aircraft was shot down. Emboldened by the fact that one of their enemy's aircraft had shown itself vulnerable, a few brave Iraqi pilots spent more time each day fine-tuning their "aerial chicken games." They pushed the rules of engagement envelope by flying as close to the restricted zone as possible. No one in the US Forces was surprised because few expected Iraqi dictator Saddam Hussein to honor the cease fire unless it was strictly monitored and enforced by US and other coalition forces. These daily aerial monitoring events and other activities ensured that I, as the CENTAF Public Affairs/ Protocol officer worked seven days a week, twelve to fifteen hours a day with a two-person staff, a male Technical Sergeant and female first Lieutenant with two years of military service. Specifically, I worked with the US Army Protocol and Public Affairs divisions as the Air Force's primary event planner. I also helped coordinate how and when senior US and Saudi military officers came together to meet and socialize.

During my time in Dhahran, I was always aware that I was in a combat zone. Danger could break out at any moment, despite the formal cease-fire and No Fly Zone enforcement. However, I always felt prepared for my role in combat. My earliest days of service included disaster preparedness and combat training, and I had learned how to use and fire a 38-caliber and a 9-mm handgun. As another part of my wartime preparation, I learned how to sit for hours wearing chemical protective body gear and how to seal properly a gas mask while stating my name and social security number in a chamber filled with gas. By the time I deployed for Desert Storm, I had become reacquainted with these skills, skills that could save my life in a real combat zone. While I frequently contemplated the possibility of face-to-face combat, I was not afraid, nor were those around me. This time as a senior captain, African American female, I remembered that I had to set a positive example especially since I would be very visible as this General's official spokesperson.

I was in good health when I arrived in Saudi Arabia. Military officers had to be especially diligent in keeping in the best of health because they had to set examples for those who worked for them. A few dramatic environmental events challenged my initial claim to good health upon my arrival in Saudi. First, before my leaving Eaker, I received several very painful vaccinations that were intended to help aid in the prevention of acquiring infectious diseases. I was informed that one of the injections was anthrax; a vaccination 150,000 American military men and women received when they deployed to the Southwest Asia Theater. The other vaccination was never identified or even listed in my shot records. Members of the Governing Board of the National Research Council Fulco, Liverman and Sox (2000) noted this lack of documentation about Gulf War vaccinations was not uncommon since

> ...Medical records from the Gulf War contain little information about who received vaccines, how frequently vaccines were administered, or the timing of vaccinations relative to the other putative exposure....further, existing record entries show no consistency in recording the type of vaccine (notations include "A-VaX" "Vacc A," Vacc B" and "B Vaccination."). A report by the Office of the Special Assistant for Gulf War Illness (OSAGWI, 1999) found that documents from the Gulf War indicate confusion about where or whether the vaccinations were to be recorded. (2000, p. 268)

After an eighteen-hour flight and still harboring a sore left hip and right gluteus maximus from the injections, I stepped out of a civilian 737 aircraft completely worn out and jetlagged. My body sagged as I wilted in the 125-degree furnace heat blasting up from the tarmac in Dhahran. My eyes started tearing up and tingling, and my throat began to burn as if I had swallowed hot coals. Caught up in a frenzied fit of coughing and gagging, I could barely catch my breath. I eventually discovered that the trigger for my coughing jag was oil well fire smoke wafting from Kuwait. More than six hundred Kuwaiti oil wells ignited by fleeing Iraqi troops in February 1991 were still burning in August (Drexler, McQueen Stauncher, 1994, p. 2103). The nagging, hacking cough and soreness of throat continued for several months during and after my deployment. Wanting to remain in worldwide duty condition and not be sent home early from this deployment, I only visited the military doctors in Dhahran once or twice. I had been seen by the doctors for a rash that had suddenly appeared on my legs, back, and arms; unknowingly an initial symptom of GWI and respite from the persistent nagging cough. It was suggested that the rash was most likely due to stress or an allergic reaction to the heavy starch the base laundry put in our camouflaged Battle Dress Uniforms (BDUS). Although there were many other soldiers coughing, the doctors never directly addressed the persistent coughing. I continued doing my job and after four months in Saudi Arabia, I returned to the United States and began my official multi-symptom rapid descent further into an invisible illness.

Upon my return to the United States, the persistent cough continued, and the rash was getting worse. I began to talk to other people from my installation and other military bases who had deployed during the war, asking them how they felt when they returned home. Several were experiencing the same types of health problems I was; some were experiencing worse. Some of us began to wonder if it was just the stress of combat or something else we were not being told. McFall (2000) et al. in a study outlining future costs of Gulf War veterans' health treatment costs showed that the puzzlement about the strange illnesses didn't lie only with us:

> Upon their return, 42 percent of Persian Gulf War veterans who reported health concerns, in the Department of Defense-sponsored Comprehensive Clinical Evaluation Program (N = 21,579), received a primary or secondary International Classification of Diseases, 9th Revision (ICD-9) diagnosis of "signs, symptoms, and ill-defined conditions." Among the most frequently reported symptoms for veterans with this diagnosis were fatigue (60 percent), joint pain (47 percent), headache (44 percent), memory loss (41 percent), sleep disturbance (41 percent), rash (30 percent), concentration difficulty (31 percent), depressed mood (30 percent), and muscle pain (22 percent). No distinctive "Gulf War Syndrome" with a known organic cause has been identified to explain these symptoms. Consequently, many health concerns of Persian Gulf War veterans have been characterized as "medically unexplained physical symptoms" (MUPS), a designation commonly used to describe health complaints when an underlying pathophysiological process cannot be found. (p. 70)

Illness for many people is an opportunity to pay more attention to our body signals (Anderson, Geist-Martin, 2003). Safely back in the United States, I began to feel my body talking to me in ways that it hadn't before. Suddenly, it was difficult for me to walk, run, or exercise consistently because my muscles and joints were in chronic pain. My energy level was low; I suffered bouts of recurring chronic fatigue that became more and more pronounced. My sleeping patterns became increasingly erratic. I could sleep for hours and still not feel refreshed when I began my day. I could hardly wait to leave work, go home, and fall right into bed. Inexplicably, I still attributed these health challenges and physiological changes to the high stress of my time in Saudi Arabia and the nonstop demands of my Eaker AFB job. I began to hear rumors about a strange new sickness that had affected people who went to the Gulf, but initially, I didn't believe it. It did not seem possible for a person to develop a mysterious illness simply by being deployed to another country. Thinking back over the eleven years of service, I remembered that I had mononucleosis earlier in my military career when I was stationed at Francis E. Warren AFB in Cheyenne, Wyoming in 1988. I began to question whether these symptoms I had started in Saudi Arabia and upon my return to Eaker were related to this previous illness. Perhaps, upon the onset of these problems I should have taken a short vacation or participated in a thorough post-deployment check up. Fiercely dedicated to duty, however, I went back to work immediately upon returning from Saudi Arabia. I was determined to resume my role as base spokeswoman for my wing commander.

The completion of my base's new mission was paramount, albeit final. Eaker AFB was going through a very painful base closure process for our military and their families, civilian staff, and local Blytheville and Gosnell, Arkansas communities. Eighteen months earlier the Defense Base Closure and Realignment Commission (BRAC) had selected Eaker AFB to close by December 1992. Ensuring that my nine-person Public Affairs Division maintained a strong, comprehensive publicity operation regarding the complexities of this closure caused my staff and me to work long hours. I participated in countless TV interviews, wrote speeches and newspaper opinion editorial pieces for my commander, and set up final base tours for state legislators, US congressional representatives, and senators. My health, I reasoned, would have to wait.

When I could no longer ignore the pain, erratic sleep, rash and the other symptoms, I finally began to seek medical intervention. The date to my pinning on my gold oak leaves to become a Major was coming closer, and I began to become even more secretive about my pain. I reluctantly began to get each malady individually treated by military and civilian doctors, which provided some temporary relief. Every day people decide whom to tell and not tell about their illnesses (Anderson, Geist-Martin, 2003). I was no exception. One of the biggest fears of a military officer has been found to have a health problem that could affect the ability to complete their leadership job in their military service's overall mission. From the first day of instruction, whether in the service academics, ROTC units or officer training schools, all officers learned that the collective military mission came first before family, friends, and self. The reluctance to make appointments with military doctors was the fear that going to see them too often would show up on my military record and be reviewed when I was being considered for future assignments. No military officer, especially a senior captain, wants to be tagged as a malingerer, and I hoped to transition seamlessly into the field grade officer ranks before retirement.

By the time I had formally transferred to my last duty assignment in December 1992, as the Director of Public Affairs for the Defense Equal Opportunity Management Institute at Patrick AFB, Cocoa Beach Florida the GWI symptoms attacked me with a vengeance. I started to have intense migraine headaches and daily bouts of Irritable Bowel Syndrome. Steroid treatments for my rashes were somewhat effective but caused me to gain unwanted weight, and I was almost put on the Air Force's punitive, career ending Weight Loss Program. Despite my efforts to keep my GWI invisible, I suspect others knew I was battling these illnesses. I continued seeing a variety of military doctors who diagnosed me with bursitis, tendinitis, colitis, even depression. I refused to see a therapist and a chaplain, as suggested by one military doctor because I did not feel all this sickness was made up in my head. My sergeant often assisted with meetings in the late afternoons when I was just so tired, and my body sagged with fatigue and intense pain. In 1994, I realized that I could possibly not be eligible for worldwide duty any longer, I swallowed my pride and put in my retirement papers. In 1993, when the US Department of Defense began offering military members the opportunity to retire with full benefits starting at fifteen years of service to nineteen years, I reluctantly took early retirement July 1, 1995, after sixteen years of service.

THE ABCS OF GWI: FINALLY FACING GULF WAR ILLNESS

In 1998, I went back to college to work on my terminal degree in Communications. By August 2005, I had my first full-time tenure track teaching appointment at Armstrong State University in Savannah, Georgia. It should have been the best time of my life, but my chronic muscle and joint pain had become unbearable. Severe mental fatigue made me feel as if I was living in a perpetual fog. I was keeping three calendars and was still forgetting things. The joy of landing a teaching appointment was short lived. I was finally ready to face my illness; I could not continue living in this pain by myself. I was ready to share my experiences with my family and a few close friends. Anderson, Geist-Martin (2003) suggest that telling stories about one's illness may be a "soothing medicine," especially if you tell those who are close to you (e.g., relatives, friends or even colleagues), but the level of one's willingness to disclose depends ultimately upon the person who has the illness. Telling a story about one's illness could increase the fear and stress associated with it. Sharing a personal narrative about one's illness could also ultimately change how one negotiates and renegotiates their relationships with those around they care about and others them. Ultimately the person with the illness shapes the context for the how, when or what they disclose. Anderson and Geist-Martin (2003) emphasize that

> ...people who feel victimized may shy away from full disclosure of their story because avoidance helps them deal with their feelings of stigmatization. On the other hand, warriors may feel like telling more people about their illness will help in their fight to conquer the disease. Others may find solace in inviting many people to share their experiences. (p. 135)

In 2006, through a strategic series of phone calls with friends, visits with family, and emails with former military colleagues, I finally shared my struggles and challenges with my health. I also decided that I would have to put my trust and overall health in the hands of my general family practice doctor who had been treating my maladies as I brought them to her attention. I had the first of a series of conversations with her about my military service and my suspicions that whatever was making me ill was because of my time in the desert. In 2007, she sent me to an orthopedic specialist who in turn, sent me to a local rheumatologist who conducted a series of tests. Finally, I had a diagnosis for the painful maladies that had been plaguing me since 1991; I had fibromyalgia, one of the illnesses associated with GWI. I was relieved, yet puzzled about that diagnosis. Looking back through my family's medical history, I could find no one on either side of my family who had claimed this as a familial health issue. When I started investigating my own health timeline, I looked back to when I began having symptoms of fibromyalgia and recurring respiratory problems that also had to be treated.

Eventually, I began to conduct my own empirical research about fibromyalgia and respiratory problems and ultimately discovered other veterans of the 1991 Gulf War had reported more cases of chronic medically unexplained symptoms than veterans of prior conflicts. I began to reflect on prior conversations that I had with others who returned from the Gulf and our comparisons of symptoms and illnesses. Now it was a bittersweet realization for me that these symptoms were very real and only now, in the twenty-first century, the government was talking about it. Gulf War Illness wasn't just stress-related phenomena. It wasn't just all in our heads; it was real.

In 2008, The Research Advisory Committee on Gulf War Veterans' Illnesses released a 454-page report that confirmed that GWI was not a stress induced psychological disease. The committee's findings left no doubt that GWI was genuine by determining:

> ...that Gulf War Illness is a real condition with real causes and serious consequences for affected veterans. Study after study has consistently documented this multisymptom condition in large numbers of Gulf War veterans. Research has also shown that this pattern of illness does not occur after every war and cannot be solely attributed to psychological stressors during the Gulf War. Because research studies have so compellingly demonstrated that Gulf War illness cannot be explained simply as the expected result of wartime stress, it remains the responsibility of the federal government to fully elaborate the

> source and nature of this condition, to care for affected veterans, and to prevent similar problems from happening in the future. (Gulf War Illness and the Health of Gulf War Veterans, 2008, Executive Summary)

FACING MY GULF WAR ILLNESS MAKES ME STRONGER

Over the past this twenty-five years, I have learned and lived the truth behind Friedrich Nietzsche's grim observation: "Out of life's school of war: What does not destroy me makes me stronger." As a retired military officer, I appreciate the effort veterans' related groups and advocacy organizations have done to approve policies and put legislation in place to address GWI and assist more than 250,000 veterans and their family members who are suffering from the effects of it. I have been searching for other opportunities outside of the African American church and to share my story with other military service members, families and civilians about GWI/CMI. I would like to discuss the impact of this illness on those who served in the Gulf and the future health challenges it will bring to selected members of society as they grow older. One way I plan on sharing and telling my story as a disabled Gulf War veteran is through taping an oral history of my time in the Gulf and archiving it through the Library of Congress' Veterans History Project of the American Folklore Center. This project "collects, preserves, and makes accessible the personal accounts of American war veterans so that future generations may hear directly from veterans and better understand the realities of war" (http://www.loc.gov/vets/about.html). Offering a firsthand account of one's story told on video, with photos letters or other artifacts allows the veteran to be able to tell their story in as much detail as they choose. With the publishing of my book *Marching as to War, Personal Narratives of African American Women's Experiences in the Gulf Wars,* I have learned how to tell my own story of GWI, as well as the stories of other women who shared their experiences with me through this process. It is difficult to share a personal story about an illness that occurred as a result of serving in the military and for which no cure will be likely. It is not a story that has a happy ending, yet it's a story that must be told. Tarpley (1995) noted:

> While the stories we tell are important, it is the act of telling and hearing them told that sets us free. And it is at this most vulnerable moment, at the meeting place of pain, joy and renewed hope, where we gather up the pieces of the stories that have been waiting to be told and where our voices--although changing--are clear and strong enough for the telling... (p. 2).

I am free now and strong enough to tell my story. While I am proud of the service I gave to my country, I know it continues to cost me something. My GWI is invisible to most. I make sure that I continue to eat right, have a lighter regimen of physical exercise and take the multitude of medications and supplemental vitamins that I now receive because of the treatments for GWI related illnesses. On those days where I cannot write because of severe cognitive difficulties, I incorporate other activities or take the opportunity to relax. I utilize several calendars to make sure I get to my appointments, faculty meetings, and other commitments on time. Due to GWI, my livelier, Type A personality has been forced to settle down and now I must pick and choose strategically how best to maneuver through my day. Finally, at the end of even my worst day, I will always remember, "the soldier, above all other people, prays for peace, for he (she) must suffer and bear the deepest wounds and scars of war" (MacArthur, 1962, para. 25).

REFERENCE

Anderson, Geist-Martin (2003). "Narratives and Healing: Exploring one family's story of cancer survivorship." *Health Communication*, 15(2), 133–143.

Collins, P. (2000). *Black Feminist Thought.* (second edition). New York and London: Routledge.

Committee on Government Reform and Oversight. *Gulf War Veterans' Illnesses House Report,* 105–388. US Publishing Office, 1997.

Cooper, A. (1892). *A Voice From the South*. Xenia, Ohio: The Aldine Printing House.

Desnoyers-Colas, E. (2014). *Marching as to War: Personal Narratives of African American Women's Experiences in the Gulf Wars.* Lanham, MD: University Press of America.

Douglas MacArthur. Duty, Honor, Country West Point Speech, 1962 http://www.americanrhetoric.com/speeches/douglasmacarthurthayeraward.html

Draxler, R., McQueen, J., and Studner B. (1994). "An evaluation of air pollutant exposures due to the 1991 Kuwait Oil Fires using a Lagrangian Model." *Atmospheric Environment*, 28, (13), 97–2210.

Fulco, C., Liverman, C., and Sox, H. (2000) *Gulf War and Health Volume 1. Depleted Uranium, Sarin, Pyridostigmine Bromide, Vaccines.* Washington, DC: National Academy Press.

Haley, R., Charuvastra, E., Shell W, Buhner D, Marshall W., Biggs, M., Hopkins S,, Wolfe G, Vernino S. (Feb 2013). "Cholinergic autonomic dysfunction in veterans with Gulf War illness: confirmation in a population-based sample." *AMA Neurol.* 70, 2,191–200. doi: 10.1001/jamaneurol.2013.596.

Hooks, b. (1989). *Talking Back: Thinking Feminist, Thinking Black.* Boston: South End Press.

Hudson, N. (2015). "When family narratives conflict: An autoethnography of my mother's secrets." *Journal of Family Communication*, 15,113–129.

Institute of Medicine (2014). "Chronic Multi symptom Illness in Gulf War veterans." *National Academic Press.*

Institute of Medicine (2010). *Gulf War and Health: Volume 8.* National Academies Press.

Kreps, G. (2012). "Health Communication inquiry and health outcomes." *Communicao Sociedade Numero Especia,* l, 11–22.

Library of Congress. *Veterans History Project*. http://www.loc.gov/vets/about.html

McFall, M. (2005). "Predicting costs of Veterans Affairs health care in Gulf War: veterans with medically unexplained physical symptoms." *Military Medicine*, 170, 1, 70–75.

Peterson, E. (2002). *The Message: The bible in contemporary language*. Colorado Springs: Nav Press.

Pierce, P. (May 2005). "Monitoring the Health of Persian Gulf War Women." *Military Medicine* 170, 5,349.

Reardon, S. (January, 2015). "The insurmountable Gulf." *Nature*, 517, 8.

Research Advisory Committee on *Gulf War Illness and the Health of Gulf War Veterans.* Department of Veterans Affairs, 2008.

Rose, T. (2003). *Longing to Tell: Black Women Talk About Sseuality and Intimacy*, New York: Farrar, Straus and Giroux.

Shriver, T., and Waskul, D. (2006). "Contested Illness: Managing the uncertainties of Gulf-War Illness." *Symbolic Interaction*, 29, 4, 465–486.

Sparkes, A.C. (2000). "Autoethnography and narratives of self: Reflections on criteria in action." *Sociology of Sport Journal*, 17, 21–43.

Spieldenner, A. (Winter 2014). "Statement of ownership: An autoethnography of living with HIV." *The Journal of Men's Studies*, 22, 1, 12–27.

Stern, D. (2015). "Engaging Autoethnography: Feminist voice and narrative intervention." *Women and Language*, 38, 1, 83–102.

Tarpley, N. (Ed). (1995). *Testimony: Young African Americans on Self Discovery and Black Identity.* Boston: Beacon Press Book

US Department of Veterans Affairs. "Gulf War Illness." https://www.vets.gov/health-care/health-conditions/conditions-related-to-service-era/gulf-war/

US Department of Veterans Affairs. "War Related Illness and Injury Study Center."http://www.warrelatedillness.va.gov/

Chapter Nine

Complicit in Concealing Illness

Black Women, Beauty, Identity, and Breast Cancer

Annette Madlock Gatison

It is a peculiar sensation, this double consciousness, this sense of always looking at one's self through the eyes of others, of measuring one's soul by the tape of a world that looks on in amused contempt and pity. One ever feels her [sic] twoness,—an American, a Negro; two souls, two thoughts, two unreconciled strivings, two warring ideals in one dark body whose dogged strength alone keeps it from being torn asunder.

(Du Bois, *The Souls of Black Folk*)

I did not recognize myself in the mirror. My caramel complexion was full of splotches, and I had dark circles around my eyes. It was 2003, my first occurrence of breast cancer; I had six more rounds of chemotherapy to go. Like any other day, I brushed my teeth, washed my face, and combed my hair. But this day was different. This day it started; the hair loss I was warned about had started. A comb, a brush, then, just my hand—my hair just came out. As each strand released from my scalp, it hurt, and I cried. The natural hair that I had come to love long before loving your natural hair was a movement would be styled in almost shoulder length curly two strand twists. I contemplated grabbing a pair of scissors to cut my remaining hair off myself, but I could not bring myself to do it. That hair, my hair, as I knew it would be no more. I shared this devastating news with my pastor. She suggested we have a special ceremony to say goodbye as the remaining curly strands of black hair were cut from my head. One of the sisters from my church was a hairstylist and owned a salon. This was a close knit church family, and I was open to the idea. It was a special time; no other clients were in the shop that day; there was just the three of us in prayer and tears as my hair fell to the floor. I had no idea who this person in the mirror was. It did not look like me. It did not feel like me. Wigs, hats, scarves, and make-up all played a part in trying to camouflage the physical changes to my body. But, how long could I keep these physical changes to myself?

It took three years and the help of an African hair braider to grow my hair back to a healthy state. It was not the same pre chemo therapy hair texture, but I was no longer bald, blotchy, tired, or weak. *They* told me, they being the medical professionals, that my risk of getting breast cancer again was minimal if I took the drug Tamoxifen for five years. Listening to this advice, I completed the cut, poison, and burn process a.k.a. lumpectomy, chemotherapy, and radiation. I began taking the daily dose of Tamoxifen in pill form and began to live my new normal.

Then, it happened again.

Technically what *they* said was true. That particular form of breast cancer did not return. The second occurrence was the opposite breast and another type of aggressive breast cancer. Yet again, my life was on the line. Yet again, I was concerned about how to keep this secret as I worked to maintain my lively hood. I was also in fear of the physical changes. I did not want to lose my hair *again*, go through the blotchy skin *again*, or gain weight *again*. Yes, some women do gain weight rather than lose weight as some of the steroids cause weight gain and bloating. The steroids are used to help you tolerate the cancer drugs flowing through your veins killing off any fast growing cells in the body.

I was afraid and wanted to hide.

I did what *they* told me to do. I followed the rules. Cut. Poison. Burn. Yet, she was back.

The weak, tired, bald, blotchy, breast cancer patient was back. The woman who sat in her hair stylists chair and watched her hair fall to the floor was back. This time my hair loss was more traumatic for my Dominican hairdresser than it was for me. Unlike her, I knew what was coming. She is the one who shed the tears. In essence, she cried for me. My stylist could not bring herself to cut my hair off. It was another stylist who happened to be the salon owner who eventually did the deed, the cutting of my hair. I silently prayed to myself, no big fanfare or ceremony this time.

In this very superficial world, looks are so important. Even if you are not healthy the façade of health and beauty are significant at work, for family, friends, and life in general. The western American/US culture is not about looking at and caring for the sick and aged. The cultural norms of beauty, youth, and superficiality are also part of the work place. Which always brings me to a fearful place in which I ask the following questions: How much do I share about my health and wellness? As a university professor, I am always on display. Will my job and or career be put in jeopardy? How long can I hide my illness? Higher education is not immune from these biases against the differently abled, raced, or gendered so these questions must be asked. At the end of each semester, students are asked to rate their professors via a survey instrument or course evaluation. It is well documented that female faculty of color are held to a different standard on these types of survey instruments[1] and have different experiences and interactions with students due to racial bias and identity negotiation in the classroom (Harlow, 2003).

Some students are not very kind on those opinion surveys. As a black professor, I am judged harshly by some on those opinion surveys on things that should have no bearing on the quality of my teaching. What I am wearing and my hair should not be of any significance—but a large black woman with braids and wearing a suit is intimidating. These were actual comments from previous course evaluations. This is an indication that even when you are presumed to be healthy and somewhat conforming to the professional norm your appearance is communicating something. Opie and Phillips (2015) conducted three experimental studies that examined the influence of race, Afrocentric hairstyles versus Eurocentric hairstyles, and perceptions of dominance and professionalism in the workplace. In each of the studies, they used images of white and black women in business suits with Afrocentric or a straight Eurocentric hairstyle and concluded in all three studies that choice in hairstyle matters. In my case trying to hide illness resulted in less face-to-face time with students. I thought less interpersonal interaction would not be as stressful. Having to "justify my existence" under healthy circumstances creates its own set of stressors and hostile spaces.

So I taught online courses and held virtual office hours. As I reflect back, there was not much self-care in this compromise. Not much self-care at all in this online teaching space and not much rest. Online courses are more work than traditional face-to-face courses. However, I was not burdened with the psychological trauma of explaining why I looked different for those who actually noticed nor would I have to concern myself with course evaluations that commented on my looks and not the actual course content or course delivery. Choosing this compromise was about financial security, which is also about self-care in the short-term. I needed to make sure I would have health insurance throughout the duration of this illness and treatment plan as well as the ability to pay my mortgage, student loan, and other life expenses. After the second lumpectomy, part of my treatment plan was once again chemotherapy. I was on a weekly to bi-weekly, six- to eight-hour chemo drip (intravenous) for a number of months. I graded papers, talked to students, and facilitated online courses. I was trying to hide the physical impact of my illness as much as I could. Then, there was just no point in hiding because for some of us life goes on. I have to say this as some of the women I met transitioned to the next life—DEATH—and there is no need to hide any longer—LIFE. So, you come out of hiding in honor of the women who are not with us on this plane of existence. Blotchy skin and dark circles can be hidden with makeup, and hats and scarves are my friends.

During this time, the health care professionals did not tell me that one of the intravenous drugs—Taxotere—could possibly leave me totally bald, partially bald, or with extremely thin hair. However, I am considered one of the lucky ones. Some of my hair grew back, but once again it was very different from the hair I started with—very thin, sparse, and weak. While I use my ability to accessorize with wigs, hats, and scarves to my advantage, I still do not truly know the person looking back at me in the mirror. I am still trying to embrace this pink identity. That of a two-time breast cancer survivor.

BACKGROUND

The standards of beauty that are socially constructed for African American/black women be they Eurocentric or Afrocentric (Byrd and Tharpe, 2014; Djaine, 2009; Spellers and Moffitt, 2010) come with an expectation to be upheld and does not overwhelmingly include being breastless, bald, and chronically ill[2]. Black female breast cancer survivors have an increased burden of conformity to these standards, which based on the level of performance can be both an asset and a burden. Please know that I am not advocating for or advancing the idea that one should walk around "looking sickly," "bent over," and "sad faced" or performing whatever ones visual representation of illness might be. However, as a black woman when you do not "look sick" perceptions of the severity of illness or need for help are altered (Madlock Gatison, 2016).

Therefore, when it comes to visual representations of wellness and beauty as asset or burden, one has to think twice. As a probable asset, there is some truth to the idea that if you look good, you just might feel a little better. The burden is in that it creates another type of identity and layer of invisibility as it pertains to the existence of breast cancer or illness[3] in black women. This is an area of inquiry that receives relatively little attention in the current health communication scholarship. Although there is a preponderance of health communication research, it rarely addresses in depth black women's challenges to dominant cultural definitions of womanhood and beauty when it comes to the impact of illness, visible or invisible on the self or others. With cancer being listed as a type of disability and chronic illness, it bears repeating the widely known fact that African American women have a lower incidence rate of breast cancer when compared to white or Asian women in the United States however; they are still burdened with a higher mortality rate than other racial groups (Daly and Olopade, 2015).

When addressing breast cancer in black women, one must remember that it is not only the biochemical component of the disease that renders it hazardous to one's health, it is also the cultural and environmental factors that should be considered (Fisher Collins, 2006; Torres, 2009). This chapter extends a report from a previous study, The Pink and The Black Project (PABP), that looked at how the trifecta of strength emanating from the rhetoric of breast cancer warrior metaphors, Christian faithtalk, and the strong black woman ideology influenced African American female breast cancer survivors perceptions of self and how others perceived them (Madlock Gatison, 2016). The focus here will be on visual representations of beauty and complicit invisibility and perceptions.

I use personal narrative and standpoint theory to investigate the instances when social and cultural norms call for me, a black/African American female breast cancer survivor and other survivors to be complicit in concealing our illness through appearance. Personal narrative as the methodological framework is used to examine the performativity of disclosing illness identity. According to Langellier (1999, p. 128 as cited in Defenbaugh, 2013) "approaching personal narrative as performance requires theory, which takes context as seriously as it does text....[and] examining the cultural production and reproduction of identities and experience." As an African American woman, standpoint theory provides the necessary lens for an African American female perspective for that context. As standpoint theory argues "US black women have access to the experiences that accrue to being both black and female, an alternative epistemology used to rearticulate a black women's standpoint should reflect the convergence of both sets of experiences. Race and gender may be analytically distinct, but in black women's everyday lives, they work together (Collins, 2000, p. 269)." Narrative and standpoint are what is needed to legitimize the experiences of black women and not the continued citation of scholarly texts that do not include our experiences.

> When we fail to see black women as agents of history with a dualistic structure that incorporates both an ethnic community and an oppressive society, we make errors and paint partial portraits that must be corrected, revised, and reshaped as our knowledge, insight, and critical skills grow. (Gilkes, 1989, p. 574)

It is my hope that this chapter becomes a part of the corrected, revised, and reshaped knowledge and insight into black women breast cancer survivors as it pertains to sociocultural norms that influence identity and representations of illness and wellness. Noted scholar Cheryl Townsend Gilkes asserts that writings of such scholars as Paula Giddings, Deborah White, Jacqueline Jones, and Dorothy Sterling advocate that the letter and the spirit of African American women's experiences cannot be contained within one disciplinary boundary (Gilkes, 1989, p. 574) therefore this work draws upon sources both within and outside of health communication scholarship.

Historical In "Visibility" of Black Women's Illness

Diane Price Herndol[4] (1995) in her work *The Invisible (Invalid) Woman* found a lack of historical literature that acknowledged the history of African American female illness. She noted that even in the twentieth-century writings of scholars such Barbara Ehrenreich and Deirdre English, Robin and John Haller, Carol Smith Rosenberg, Mary Poovey, and Elain Showalter the majority of the illness narrative is solidly white and middle class. However, Herndol also noted that nineteenth-century narratives about African American women written by African American women included some discussion of illness however it was presented in a way that kept strength at the forefront as a means of defusing the racist commentary of the time. Herndol also acknowledges that the medical writing along with the historical and critical accounts of slave and free black women did not write about black women's illness factually. Even in nineteenth-century writings, one had to be white and upper class to suffer from illness (Herndol, 1995, p. 554).

The work of Harriet Washington (2006) *Medical Apartheid the Dark History of Medical Experimentation on Black Americans from Colonial Times to the Present,* provides a historical look at illness and medicine that for some might help to shed some additional light as to the performance of hiding illness and silence by black women when it comes to their own health. In recent years the visibility of black women's health has been researched across disciplines as it relates to access to health care, affordability of health care, quality of health care, and sociocultural influences such as religion and family (Madlock Gatison, 2016, pp. xvi-xvii); however, the research on identity and breast cancer in black women has been scant.

Identity

Embracing the identity of breast cancer survivorship for some can be burdensome and filled with trepidation. I began this chapter with the quote by Du Bois because it speaks to the issue of identity, the burden and the fear along with some excerpts from my personal cancer journals. Gilkes (Du Bois, 1903/2012, Afterword), a noted scholar of Du Bois's work, writes specifically about Du Bois's analysis of African American women's roles and activities as well as Du Bois's acknowledgment of black women's importance to culture. Our identity matters, our health matters, our wellness matters; past present, and future.

For black women, Du Bois's text concerns itself with the many lenses by which we might view ourselves and in which others might view us. Part of my early resistance to embracing this pink identity was to not talk about it. I found this to be a common response to PABP participants. Personally, during my first occurrence with breast cancer, I did not even tell my own mother until I could no longer physically hide the effects of treatment or the distress in my voice. I did my best to remain silent and always look my best in all places and public spaces. Content to move and proceed through daily life as a fully complete, able, and well person.

In contemplating this additional identity of a breast cancer survivor, as an individual with a chronic illness, as an African American woman whose body has turned in on itself arose a conflicted and complex persona. And within this complex persona standing guard is the conflict, the "double consciousness," or as Finley (2010) explicates Du Bois's work, it is about the competing and often conflicting set of ideas located in or on the bodies of people who have experienced hegemonic existences (p. 399). In the realm of breast cancer, the hegemonic existence is in the constant comparison, narrative, and research centered on the survivor who is representatively white, middle or upper class.

Finley (2010) goes on to state that Du Bois's double consciousness theory "means that black people's experience of hegemony in the United States split their consciousness regarding the body. The resulting sociocultural construction of the body in which the conflict was located reflected this split, the negation of the Blackbody [*including the hair and breasts*], and at the same time the valorization of the culture of oppression" [*the embracing of a European aesthetic or standard of beauty as the normalized body*] is burdensome and detrimental to black women who have survived breast cancer. Using the warrior metaphors so prevalent in western culture during wellness we are literally in the fight for our black lives mentally and physically every day as we combat institutional and structural "isms." Now one must add to this the fight against illness an invisible illness, in this case, breast cancer. A disease that does not always show itself or the side effects from treatment.[5]

Complicity

What does it mean to be complicit? The simple denotative definition of complicit according to Merriam-Webster.com is "helping to commit a crime or do wrong in some way." So what does it meant to be complicit in concealing illness, particularly for black women? I contend that it means that we remain silent when we are hurting both mentally and physically. This "wrong doing" is done in the simplest of ways such as not seeking medical attention in a timely fashion, taking on too many responsibilities, and/or not asking for help when needed, and of course not getting proper rest, nutrition, or exercise. But this complicity and concealment of illness is helped along by the social and cultural norms that surround expectations for black women's strength and standards for appearance. I am guilty of being complicit, not just through my silence as discussed earlier, but also through embracing the strong black woman identity even though it was out of necessity.

Fashioned Survivor

Women who have been diagnosed with breast cancer or are survivors of the disease are encouraged to manage appearance-related side effects of cancer treatment such as chemotherapy induced alopecia (loss of hair from the head, eyebrows, even eyelashes in varying degrees) and surgical mastectomy (Zoretti, 2015), which is the removal of one or both breasts. The loss of hair and breasts are not ambiguous. They are very obvious and are the cause of stress and anxiety (Williams 2008) for some women and challenge the sense of self, identity, and womanhood (Henderson, 2014; Thompson, 2009; Torres, 2009). Depending on the severity of the cancer and the length and toxicity of the chemotherapy one's hair does not always grow back the same if the hair grows back at all.

When these losses are visually obvious, and there are no other visual indicators of illness they call into question one's sanity/mental health or sexual orientation by others. For example, when I hurriedly left the safety of my home and inadvertently forgot to cover my shiny bald head I overheard comments in a public space such as: *"What woman in her right mind would walk around with a head looking like that?" "She must be gay." "You know it takes all kinds."* I was exposed, but my illness was not visible. These comments were problematic and the cause of much added mental anguish during this time. As one who would never appear in public without something to cover my head, there was a feeling of stupidity that I had forgotten to do this, as I knew the consequences of being a bald black woman in public. I attributed the forgetfulness on chemobrain (post chemotherapy cognitive impairment) and the fact that it was too hot for a wig or hat. The visual representations of the fashioned survivor promote an image that is according to Ozum Ucok (2007) desirable and beautiful even when a person is sick a standard of beauty that is complicated for African American Women.

When It Comes to Our Hair

Black women's hair has been the topic of discussion for centuries from the early slave narratives to the politics of the twenty-first century (Byrd and Tharps, 2014; Spellers and Moffitt, 2010). From wearing it in it styles that are conducive to the hairs' natural curl pattern; to straightening the hair with chemicals or heat; and adding hair as in the form of wigs, braided extensions, and weaves. There is much versatility to black hair and hair styling options. This versatility can be imagined on what some might call a continuum starting with the natural/kinky coils and curls with an unapologetically African standard for beauty to the Eurocentric beauty standard for hair long and straight. Through the course of time, the African-centered standard for beauty has gained a greater acceptance with black women embracing natural hairstyles, however, in the larger majority social structure, the standard of beauty for body and hair is still Eurocentric.

I was surprised to find this Eurocentric beauty ideal reinforced in a black church with the use of Biblical passages such as: *If a woman has long hair, it is a glory to her; for her hair is given to her for a covering* (1 Corinthians 11:15). I call attention to this based on a sermon I recently heard preached from the pulpit of a Pentecostal/Sanctified church. Yes, on a twenty-first-century Sunday morning. This message caught me off guard as I had never in my experience as a Christian heard this passage of scripture preached to admonish women for wearing short hair as it was "masculine" and "other things." However, I thought that maybe I was being overly sensitive because it was during this time that I was also dealing with therapeutic side effects of lingering toxins in my body that caused thin, weakened hair. I had to confer with another parishioner who was also a black female breast cancer survivor to make sure that I heard the sermon correctly; I had. By this time, I had learned that hair is coded, and the style one chooses to wear can send many messages from socioeconomic status to sexuality. But, I had never attended a Pentecostal Sanctified church before and had to learn that the role and dress code for women was gender specific and came with performative rules (Gilke, 1986; Alexander, 2011).

Hair as Performance

"If you don't feel good about your hair, you don't feel good about yourself, and thus you don't feel good about others" (White, 2010, p. 23). There is a heteronormativity to hairstyles, and within the black community, baldness is not a female gendered womanly norm (Lane-Steele, 2011; Prince, 2009). In L.H. Stallings (2010) work *Coming Out Natural: Dreaded Desire Sex Roles and Cornrows,* the author discusses the meaning of hairstyles and their functions. For example, the physicality of a shaved bald head is masculine "whereas relaxed hair extensions and braids seem to be explicitly tied to feme identification and bald, short crop cuts and cornrows function as Butch aesthetics twists then cornrows and dreadlocks appear to be androgynous or alternative aesthetics in black queer communities" (p. 377).

When I saw someone with hair that was natural or relaxed, short and cropped, long straight, curly or colored blond, brown, red, green or purple, it never occurred to me to question their sanity or sexuality. Well, there was a time I might have questioned the green or purple hair, but times have changed. However, should I ever forget to wear my hair covering while regrouping from the side effects of chemotherapy one thing I know for sure; that it will be my sanity and sexuality that will be questioned. This experience draws closer to my attention the presumption of deviance experienced by my queer brothers and sisters; as both mental illness and queerness are framed as deviant in the broader society. I can only draw from my childhood experience pre-relaxer days when the press[6] and curl[7] is what you would get. My maternal grandmother had a good friend who would do our hair. It was not until I was much older that it was explained to me that he was a gay man. I could see that he was a man, I say that because literally, he looked like Ving Rhames's character in the movie *Holiday Heart*, but like my grandmother, he dressed in old flowery house dresses. Nothing outrageous or flamboyant just what I would call grandma clothes. But, it was still all about the hair, Holiday, my grandmother's friend, could handle those Marcel irons like nothing I had ever seen.

Rites of Passage

For some of us, we learned at an early age about who does and does not have good hair, and what makes up good hair. We even learned that if you do not have good hair how to get it via a hard press (with good hair you might just need a warm comb or nothing at all), a good relaxer and when you get a little older wigs and weaves. Shauntae Brown White (2010) discusses the politics of natural hair versus relaxed hair and what is considered normative in the black community as it relates to what some see as a young girls rite of passage or coming of age in the black community that move to "the big girl's chair" (p. 23).

It is necessary to bring up beauty shops and the "big girl's chair" as this was and still is the space where researchers and practitioners go to spread the breast cancer awareness message, find out about attitudes and screening behaviors among black women (Forte, 1995; Sadler et. al., 2007). With this knowledge, you would think that the American Cancer Society's *Look Good Feel Good* classes would have a better selection of makeup and wigs suitable for African American women. Unfortunately, this was not the case as reported by ten of the women who participated in the PABP focus group (Madlock Gatison, 2016) that attended the Look Good Feel Good sessions in the past.

Sociocultural standards of beauty call for African American women to conceal the illness of breast cancer. A breast cancer survivor who is working through a temporary or sustained period of baldness, changes in hair texture and length after treatment will not find the cultural norms as a space to relax. The burden to maintain one's coif and deliver an appearance of wellness is expected. In order to perform a good look, all of the strategies that one embraced for hair care have to be renegotiated and relearned. It is possible that the hair you had is no longer what you will end up with. I found this to be a struggle as one would think wearing a wig would be easy, but for me, it was not. I found wigs to be problematic; it was much easier to wear a hat during times of baldness and extremely short hair. After a certain amount of time I tried a variety of fixes from braid or twist extensions, weaves, and back to wigs and hats. This is the only way I can say it, my hair is just not the same. Discussions with the PABP participants would also come back to our hair. Hair is a significant part of a breast cancer survivor's identity gay or straight.

When we think about these components in terms of breast cancer and black women's health they are different than the experiences of white and other women of color. These differences can be seen in the early media images that shape breast cancer culture and pink ribbon rhetoric that call for white women to be strong and hopeful. Which differs for black women as the idea of strong black womanhood and faith are prescribed tools that determine how we are to act during times of tribulation and trauma, even illness. There are also in-group differences within the community of black women that shape our material reality, as there are socioeconomic and educational differences that are significant within a healthcare context but one constant remains: we all fight against the controlling image that stereotypes us as strong black women even in a sea of pink ribbons (Madlock Gatison, 2016).

As African-American women, we are masters of the mask (Beauboeuf-Lafonatant, 2009). We learn to mask early from the embodiment of strength be it mental or physical to the changing of appearance and how we wear our hair. We are weaving in and out of identities to manage the expectations that we have for ourselves or that are imposed by others. Even in illness, chronic illness we are negotiating our identities we must know how to disclose or remain silent. There are times when we must be complicit in concealing our illness because the ramifications of telling can hold serious consequences from loss of job to loss of relationships.

I am guilty of being complicit in concealing a chronic illness. In the early days, I never said a word I kept breast cancer to myself until I could not hide it anymore. I wore hats, wigs, and makeup to hide the blotchiness and other changes in my skin tone that resulted from chemotherapy. According to some even then I did not look sick. And to quote a church member "girl you don't look like what you been through." I might not look like it, but it sure feels like it.

REFERENCES

Alexander, E. (2011). *Black Fire: One Hundred Years of African American Pentecostalism.* Downers Grove, IL: IVP Academics.

Byrd, A. D. and Tharps, L. L. (2014). *Hair story: Untangling the roots of black hair in America. Revised and updated.* New York, NY: St. Martin's Griffin.

Collins, P. H. (2000). *Black feminist thought: Knowledge, consciousness, and the politics of empowerment (2nd ed).* New York, NY: Routledge.

Daly, B., and Olopade, O. I. (2015, January 13). "Race, Ethnicity, and the Diagnosis of Breast Cancer." *JAMA: Journal of the American Medical Association.* pp. 141–142.

Davis, O. I. (2008). "A Visitation from the Foremothers: Black Women's Healing Through a 'Performance of Care'—From African Diaspora to the American Academy." *Women's Studies In Communication*, *31*(2), 175–185.

Defenbaugh, N. L. (2013). "Revealing and concealing ill identity: A performance narrative of IBD disclosure." *Health Communication, 28, 159–169.* Doi: 10.1080/10410236.2012.666712.

Djanie, A. (2009). "The black woman and the beauty myth." *New African*, (488), 60–61.

Du Bois, W. E. B. (1903, 2012). *The souls of black folk*. Signet Classics Edition. New York, NY: Penguin Group.

Finley, S. C. (2010). "Two warring ideals, one dark body: Hegemony, duality, and temporality of the black body and African-American religion." In Regina E. Spellers and Kimberly R. Moffitt (Eds.) *Blackberries and redbones: Critical articulations of black hair/body politics in Africana communities.* Cresskill, NJ: Hampton Press.

Fisher Collins, C. (2006). *African American women's health and social issues*. Westport, CT: Praeger.

Forte, D. A. (1995). "Community-based breast cancer intervention program for older African American women in beauty salons." *Public Health Reports*, *110*(2), 179.

Gallia, K., and Pines, E. (2009). "Narrative identity and spirituality of African American churchwomen surviving breast cancer survivors." *Journal of Cultural Diversity*, *16*(2), 50–55.

Gilkes, C. T. (1989). "Dual Heroisms and double burdens: Interpreting Afro-American women's experience and history." *Feminist Studies,* 15(3), pp. 573–590.

Gilkes, C. T. (1986). "The Role of Women in the Sanctified Church." *Journal of Religious Thought*, *43*(1), 24.

Harlow, R. (2003). "Race doesn't matter but. . .: The effect of race on professors' experiences and emotion management in the undergraduate college classroom." *Social Psychology Quarterly*, 66(4), 348–363.

Henderson, C. E. (2014). "AKA: Sarah Baartman, The Hottentot Venus, and Black Women's Identity." *Women's Studies*, *43*(7), 946–959. doi:10.1080/00497878.2014.938191.

Herndol, D. P. (1995/2010). "The invisible (invalid) woman: African-American Women, Illness, and nineteenth-century narrative." *Women's Studies, 24(6), 553–572.* doi http://dx.doi.org/10.1080/00497878.1995.9979081.

Johnson, J. C., Gamst, G., Meyers, L. S., Arellano-Morales, L., and Shorter-Gooden, K. (2016). "Development and validation of the African American Women's Shifting Scale (AAWSS)." *Cultural Diversity And Ethnic Minority Psychology*, *22*(1), 11–25. doi:10.1037/cdp0000039.

Lomax, T. A. (2016). "Technology of Living." *Black Scholar*, *46*(2), 19–32.

Kundrat, A. L. and Nussbaum, J. F. (2003). "The impact of invisible illness on identity and contextual age across the life span." *Health Communication, 15(3), 331–347.*

Lane-Steele, L. (2011). "Studs and protest-hypermasculinity: the tomboyism within black lesbian female masculinity." *Journal of Lesbian Studies*, 15, 480–492. Doi:10.1080/10894160.2011.532033.

Lester, N. A. (2010). "Of wigs and weaves, locks and fades: A personal political hair story." In Regina E. Spellers and Kimberly R. Moffitt (Eds.) Blackberries and redbones: Critical articulations of black hair/body politics in Africana communities. Cresskill, NJ: Hampton Press.

Madlock Gatison, A. (2016). *Health communication and breast cancer among Black women: culture, identity, spirituality, and strength.* Lanham, MD: Lexington Books.

Merriam-Webster.com online dictionary http://www.merriam-webster.com/dictionary/complicit

Opie, T. R. and Phillips, K. W. (2015). "Hair penalties: the negative influence of Afrocentric hair on ratings of Black women's dominance and professionalism." *Frontiers in Psychology*, 6, 1311, www.frontiersin.org. doi: 10.3389/fpsyg.2015.01311.

Personal Care Products Council Foundation, The. (2015). *Look Good Feel Better.* Retrieved from http://lookgoodfeelbetter.org.

Prince, A. (2009). *The politics of black women's hair*. London, Ontario: Insomniac Press.

Sadler, G. R., Ko, C. M., Cohn, J. A., White, M., Weldon, R., and Wu, P. (2007). "Breast cancer knowledge, attitudes, and screening behaviors among African American women: the Black cosmetologists promoting health program." *BMC Public Health*, 757–8. doi:10.1186/1471–2458–7-57

Settles, I., Pratt-Hyatt, J., and Buchanan, N. (2008). "Through the lens of race: black and white women's perceptions of womanhood." *Psychology of Women Quarterly*, *32*(4), 454–468 15.

Spellers, R. E. and Moffitt, K. R. (Eds.) (2010). *Blackberries and Redbones: Critical Articulations of Black Hair/Body Politics in Africana Communities.* Creskill, NJ: Hampton Press.

Stallings, L. H. (2010). "Coming out natural: Dreaded desire sex roles and cornrows." In Regina E. Spellers and Kimberly R. Moffitt (Eds.) *Blackberries and redbones: Critical articulations of black hair/body politics in Africana communities.* Cresskill, NJ: Hampton Press.

Tate, S. A. (2009). *Black Beauty: Aesthetics, Stylization, Politics*. Farnham, Surrey, England: Routledge.

Tate, S. (2007). "Black beauty: Shade, hair and anti-racist aesthetics." *Ethnic & Racial Studies*, *30*(2), 300–319. doi:10.1080/01419870601143992.

Thompson, C. (2009). "Black Women, Beauty, and Hair as a Matter of Being." *Women's Studies*, *38*(8), 831–856. doi:10.1080/00497870903238463.

Torres, B. A. (2009). "Dangerous Identities: Femininity and Breast Cancer in Latin America." *Journal of Latino-Latin American Studies (JOLLAS)*, *3*(4), 1–12.

Ucok, O. (2007). "The fashioned survivor: Institutionalized representations of women with breast cancer." *Communication & Medicine (De Gruyter)*, *4*(1), 67–78. doi:10.1515/CAM.2007.008

Wesley, Y. (2009). *Black Women's Health: Challenges and Opportunities*. New York: Nova Science Publishers, Inc.

Williams, T. (2008). *Black Pain: It only looks like were not hurting*. New York, NY: Simon & Schuster, Inc.

White, S. B. (2010). "The big girl's chair: A rhetorical analysis of how Motions for Kids markets relaxers to African American girls." In Regina E. spellers and Kimberly R. Moffitt (Eds.) *Blackberries and redbones: Critical articulations of black hair/body politics in Africana communities.* Cresskill, NJ: Hampton Press.

Zoratti, J. (2015, April 2). "Visible again after breast surgery." *Winnipeg Free Press (MB)*. p. B1.

NOTES

1. See the following link for associated research: http://blogs.lse.ac.uk/impactofsocialsciences/2016/03/08/gender-bias-in-academe-an-annotated-bibliography/
2. Chronic illness in this essay is in reference to breast cancer survivors who are in or out of remission.
3. Disabled World is an online resource that provides an alphabetical list of medical conditions that are listed as invisible. http://www.disabled-world.com/info/all.php#c
4. Herndol self identifies in this work as a white woman.
5. Depending on the severity of the breast cancer will determine the type and length of treatment protocols. The standard course of treatment might include, chemotherapy, radiation, and lumpectomy (removal of the lump or mass), or mastectomy (the removal of one or both breasts). Side effects can include but are not limited to the following lymphedema, cognitive impairment, temporary or permanent loss of hair, neuropathy, and weight gain or loss.
6. A straightening comb or hot comb is a metal comb that once heated to a safe temperature is used to straighten moderate or coarse hair to create a smoother texture.
7. Marcel irons are heated to a safe temperature and used to curl the hair after it is pressed/straightened.

Chapter Ten

The Enemy at the Door

My Friend's Silent Battle against Breast Cancer

Wei Sun

There is a saying in the Chinese linguistic community: *When cancer is mentioned, one's face turns ash pale.* Perhaps the saying emerged from fear and uncertainty of the disease; because, although one in eight American women will develop breast cancer in her lifetime, statistically speaking, that woman is rarely Asian (cancer.org, 2007). Nevertheless, three out of five of my Chinese sister-friends who live in a metropolitan area were diagnosed with breast cancer within one year. Studies in recent years show an increase in breast cancer incidence among Asian women who migrated to America for a long time and have adopted western lifestyles.

In the Chinese community both in the United States and in China, I encountered many who were diagnosed with and some who passed away because of cancer. Some were relatives, and others were friends or acquaintances. The consistent element in all examples was that the news of the diagnoses was never openly discussed; people only whispered or skirted around the subject.

Crippled by the fear of cancer, many within this co-cultural group would rather ignore the disease rather than acknowledge its existence. This cultural "silent treatment" surrounding cancer adds to decreased survivorship rates and negatively impacts the relationships of cancer patients and their family members and friends (Lent, 2007; Liao et al., 2017; Nicolaisen et al., 2014; Sun and Critchfield, 2012; Waldrop et al., 2011). It prevents people from openly discussing cancer and thus prevents the delivery of effective social and emotional support for cancer patients.

It is common practice in China not to immediately inform a patient diagnosed with cancer of their condition. Instead, doctors usually engage with family members rather than the patient. Often, patients are not told of their diagnoses, and no one dares to take the responsibility of breaking the bad news. The exception occurs if the patient insists on being informed. The community around the cancer patient is so wary of discussing the illness that cancer patients end up feeling ostracized and ashamed. This isolates them from receiving the social and emotional support they need. On the other hand, health providers, family members, and friends of the patient believe that limiting discussion about the patient's diagnosis shields the patient from unnecessary psychological burdens (Sun and Critchfield, 2012). No matter how much people want to avoid the cancer topic, *the enemy is at the door,* and there must be a way to better cope with the experience.

Yijun was one of my three Chinese American sister-friends diagnosed with breast cancer within a twelve-month span. I was by her side through her death as well as her final arrangements. I was the closest to walk with her in the final stage of her life. In this study, I use analytical autoethnography to address (1) the roles in which culture impacts health communication, (2) how minority invisibility hindered the breast cancer survivorship of Yijun, (3) how the apprehension around discussing the topic of cancer obstructs the formation of relational support for cancer patients in the Chinese American community, (4) and what the cultural community and health providers can learn from the lived experience of Yijun.

INVISIBILITY, GENDER, AND HEALTH

This section reviews minority invisibility in health communication, women's invisible experiences in cancer, and challenges that hinder minority women from taking advantage of breast cancer screening. Research indicates that members of co-cultural groups are often rendered invisible within a mainstream culture (Orbe, 1998; Sun and Starosta, 2006; Sun 2007). Co-cultural groups do not belong to or share the same beliefs of a larger or dominant culture. Cancer patients belong to a co-cultural group. Like others dealing with invisibility, cancer patients experience the world differently from those who are not living with cancer. Their feelings and emotions are downplayed, ignored, or simplified. The invisible experiences are often negative, resulting in low self-esteem and demeaned existences for marginalized members of co-cultural groups (Sun and Critchfield, 2012; Madlock Gatison, 2016).

The American Cancer Society cautions that in the United States, minority members continue to bear the greatest cancer burdens (2017). Ethnic minorities' socioeconomic status influence their rate of risk for cancer. Lifestyles (smoking, exercise, nutrition, etc.), income, education, and health insurance coverage determine access to early screening/detection, treatment, and palliative care. In a study of women diagnosed with gynecological cancer, Giaconomi and his associates indicate:

> To understand the issue linked to invisibility, we must keep in mind that cancer is a disease that can be characterized, among other things, by a gap between the reality of the disease and the symptoms experienced by patients ... As such, gynecological cancer is perceived as an abstract disease, a perception that is reinforced by the description of cancer as a "silent disease" by some specialists. This remark allows us to differentiate between a woman's objective symptoms and subjective feelings, which may both belong to the sphere of invisibility. (2014, p. 797)

Several studies have examined the emotional well-being of women cancer survivors. Side effects of surgery, chemotherapy, and radiation treatments may result in the loss of hair, removal of female organs, scars, and change in body shape. All of these resulting factors often make women feel humiliated because they may feel their female identity is threatened. They may believe they are no longer meeting society's beauty standards and lose confidence that they are still physically attractive to their intimate partners (Hofmann, 2004; Giaconomi et al., 2014; Sun and Critchfield, 2012). These insecurities may lead survivors to isolate themselves from the rest of the world.

Decades of cancer research have led to decreases in cancer morbidity and mortality rates in the United States since 2000. Early screening and early diagnosis of certain type of cancer have saved lives of many people (NIH, 2017). A challenge still exists in relaying information regarding cancer screenings and cancer prevention programs to ethnic minorities. Once diagnosed with cancer, many are overwhelmed with urgent matters such as how to find credible resources for care, how to pay medical expenses, and where to find social and emotional support. Ethnic minority members may even sometimes hold cultural beliefs that prevent them from the advantages produced by research stated earlier. According to a study conducted by Frisby (2002), many African American women do not undergo mammography, an effective way to prevent breast cancer, because many of them hold negative perceptions about breast cancer, which is connected to notions of fear, impairment, and death. As compared to that of white women, the overall death rates of black women were 42 percent higher. From 2003 to 2012, white women's breast cancer mortality rates decreased significantly in all fifty states. But for black women, mortality rates decreased in only twenty-seven states (DeSantis et al., 2015).

Breast cancer is the most commonly diagnosed cancer and the leading cause of death for Asian American women. Studies show that Asian women living in the United States for more than ten years have higher breast cancer incidence rates than those who live in Asian countries and have an 80 percent higher risk than new immigrants of developing breast cancer (Gomez et al.,

2010; Luhar, 2015). Immigration, change of diet, social stresses, and environmental factors are all contributors to the higher cancer incidence rates among this group (Andreeva et al., 2007). Cultural and language barriers and lack of resources and culturally appropriate education have obstructed early diagnosis, correct decision making, and valuable social support for this group.

A recent survey of 238 Chinese cancer patients concludes that negative attitudes could increase hopelessness and other negative emotions. Increasing awareness and having a positive attitude could improve the well-being of cancer patients (Liao et al., 2017). Research has confirmed that social, emotional, and spiritual support is important to the increased quality of cancer patient recovery. Yet, few supports are available for minority women cancer patients. Minority women's voices are often silenced in society. Additionally, minority women diagnosed and living with breast cancer are much more likely to face more challenges and suffer more invisibility in the medical process of screening, diagnosis, follow-up treatment, and in receiving emotional and social support before and after the medical treatment. Cancer patients across all races and ethnicities face challenges in dealing with their pain and disharmony in life (Ferrante, Chen, and Kim, 2008; Ferrante et al., 2011; Madlock Gatison, 2016). However, minority members encounter more obstacles and disadvantages in health care systems due to minority health disparities. Madlock Gatison's (2016) black women's breast cancer research confirms that minority women suffer invisibility in equality of health care access and quality as compared to European American women. Asian American women diagnosed with breast cancer often suffer dual cultural biases since the stigma of breast cancer silences them within their ethnic groups (Luhar, 2015; Waldrop et al., 2011). In a larger societal context, lack of medical navigation and institutional support has created major problems for cancer survivorship. There is a need to address the issue and improve minority women's health in general. Raising awareness, giving voices to breast cancer patients, and sharing these patients' experiences are important in helping them fully embrace available health benefits and increase personal satisfaction in quality of life.

Previous research confirms the existence of minority invisibility in health communication, and minority women have encountered more difficulties in breast cancer. However, the lived experiences of minority women who are breast cancer patients are seldom studied. This study aims to explore the following research questions: What contributes to the invisibility of breast cancer in Chinese Americans? What has silenced the community and the patient? What implications and recommendations can be gleaned from Yijun's lived experiences in fighting and losing this battle?

THEORETICAL FRAMEWORK AND METHOD

A culture-centered approach of health communication is used as a theoretical framework. In his research on communication practices in healthcare settings, Dutta (2007) proposes that culture should be the center of the communication process and that cultural participants should co-construct the meanings in health contexts. A person's identity constructions, sense making, and life experiences are paramount in health communication. The culture-centered approach gives voice to cultural members in co-constructions of health risks faced by the community. Listening to their voices will help health institutions fully understand the problems minorities face so that in the future, policy making and intervention can be implemented in a culturally sensitive and appropriate dimension.

In this chapter, I use an analytic autoethnography method to narrate the journey my friend Yijun and I walked during her battle with cancer. Autoethnography has been used in qualitative research to describe and understand cultural experiences (Ellis and Bochner, 2006; 2000). Bochner (2012) argues that autoethnography builds a rapport relationship between the storyteller and the story listener and encourages conversations through "the heartbreaking feelings of stigma and marginalization… the therapeutic desire to face up to the challenges of life and to emerge with greater self-knowledge, the opposition to the repression of the body, the difficulty of finding the words to make bodily dysfunction meaningful" (p. 159). Analytic autoethnography not only provides personal reflections but also analyzes and generalizes data to stimulate theoretical development, refinement, and extension, and encourage further conversation. Autoethnographers can create and structure narratives in different formats. One is co-constructed narratives: this format "illustrate[s] the meanings of relational experiences, particularly how people collaboratively cope with the ambiguities, uncertainties, and contradictions about some aspect of their relations, often told about or around an epiphany" (Ellis et al., 2010, p. 349).

Epiphany is defined by Kien (2014) as:

> an identifiable moment of lived experience that one can identify as a turning point in one's understanding of oneself and one's relationship to the world. The recurring, longitudinal but unpredictable characteristic of remembering the epiphanic moment as it erupts throughout one's life leads to the description of epiphany as if it has a life of its own. Thus the epiphany compels the researcher to return to and explore that life-altering moment. (p. 578)

Kien (2014) encourages ethnographers to always return to the moments, and reexamine the epiphanies and interpret the deeper meanings behind them.

In this chapter, relational ethics is used to allow readers to understand the cultural meanings in Yijun's illness and my communication with her and others. I invite readers to co-participate as I highlight the experiences of Chinese sister-friends with culturally similar illness narratives. Yijun and I connected not only by friendship and shared Chinese values but also by a spiritual tie. She was the one who introduced me to Christianity, and that made us closer beyond a personal relationship. Pseudonyms are used to protect privacy. Validity was established through member checks with other members of the Chinese community and communication scholars to ensure validity. I leave the readers to decide if the stories speak to them about a specific culture and its members' experiences. Through the reader's interpretations of the stories of Yijun, cultural understanding could potentially be achieved which allows sense making regarding breast cancer, invisibility, and Chinese American women (Ellis and Bochner, 2002).

In this study, I use several epiphanies in the two-year journey Yijun and I walked together to try to make sense of what contributed to the invisibility of breast cancer in Chinese American communities and how we can make a change.

DATA ANALYSIS AND INTERPRETATION

Yijun was born in what the Chinese people call the *Generation of the 1950s*. This generation shared social and cultural characteristics brought forth by the historical events in their youth. They lived through famine in China as pre teens in the early 1960s. They were sent to live in poverty in the countryside during the Cultural Revolution in the decade leading up to 1976 and lived in rural areas until College Admission Examinations were reinstated in China in 1977. Yijun was admitted to college in 1977 and after graduating worked in a research institution for several years before coming to the United States in the late 1980s. Yijun was a big sister to me, the first Chinese girlfriend I made when I moved to a metropolitan area for my terminal degree studies in the late 1990s. She was also a big influence on my becoming a Christian. We frequently saw and talked to each other over the years. Her daughter, Vivi, is three years older than my daughter. Her then husband went back to China soon after I came to know the couple in 1999. He never came back to the United States until Yijun passed away. For years, Yijun was the sole provider for her family. Yijun was the youngest of her three siblings. Her brother and sister both live in China. Her parents passed away in their eighties.

Epiphany 1: Breaking the Silence, to a Selected Few

Yijun did not tell me she had cancer until a year after her diagnosis. On December 31, 2010, we sat next to each other at a New Year's Eve musical gospel concert in a Chinese Christian church. Before the concert started, I whispered to her that another mutual Chinese friend, Meihua, had recently been diagnosed with breast cancer and that two families came to church to pray for her speedy recovery that night. Yijun did not say anything that evening. Four days after, on January 3, 2011, she sent me the following email:

> Last Friday, you told me that Meihua is diagnosed with breast cancer. I did not think it was the right time and right place to share with you some information then. I think now it is the time to share it with you; we may find more time to talk later. I am diagnosed with the breast cancer, too. Please don't share this with anybody right now; I have not even told my sister and brother. God will tell me when and with whom I need to share this information. I am in very good hands and have peace in my mind…

That night I woke up after midnight due to jet lag from a trip to China one week before. I was caught completely by surprise and jumped up out of shock. My thoughts were racing: *Two pieces of bad news in less than a week! Why are so many Chinese American acquaintances getting breast cancer so suddenly?!* Reading the message, I regretted telling Yijun about Meihua's case so absent-mindedly. I wondered what she might have thought of me since she was so secretive about her illness. Was she afraid that other people would share her secret, including her siblings and me? I wanted to assure her that her secret would stay with me. So I replied to her in an email:

> I am stunned by the information, and your health is now in my prayers. I fully understand the sensitiveness of your condition; will not share the news with others.

While I advocate for open communication between cancer patients and their family members and friends, I quickly complied with her request of not telling anyone else. If I told others, I would have betrayed the friendship she entrusted to me. Sleepless for the rest of the night, I searched key words "breast cancer" online both in Chinese and English. I collected all the useful information I believed would help Yijun. I called her first thing in the morning. She said she was expecting my call that day. She recalled how, about a year previously, she felt a lump under her breast, went to the doctor, and was diagnosed with Stage 0–1 breast cancer. Nevertheless, she decided against traditional cancer treatments; instead, she chose alternative medicine, believing that herbal treatment and acupuncture would cure cancer. I asked why she hadn't told me earlier so I could help. She said she did not want to bother anyone. "I can take care of myself. So far you are only the second person to know." Then I asked her, "Why did you choose an herbal treatment from the beginning? Isn't it the first choice to have surgery, followed by chemotherapy and radiation?"

Yijun said she did not trust western medicine at all, "I did homework on cancer, and the findings are disturbing. Western medicine does more harm than good. The drugs used in chemotherapy are so aggressive that they kill both your good cells and bad cells! I am not allowing any doctor to put a knife on my body, and I am not taking any aggressive drugs!"

Epiphany 2: Decision Making on Medical Choices

Within a week of our first conversation regarding her diagnosis, Yijun underwent treatment in a naturalistic wellness center near my house. The usual routine included a vitamin C boost in the first hour to energize her body enough to receive the minimal chemotherapy treatment that followed after breakfast. She then received "light chemo" before bathing in a sauna to cleanse away any side effects the minimum chemotherapy may have caused. I accompanied her for nearly three hours for a whole cycle of the treatment. She said she needed to undergo eight of the treatments. After the session, she discussed payment with the cashier by the exit. Yijun paid $480 for one day of non-insured treatment.

I invited her to my house to rest after the treatment. I told her that I was writing a paper on cancer patients in China, and she was eager to hear about the findings and asked if it would be of benefit to cancer patients like her. I sheepishly told her, "You know my discipline is not hard science. I am looking at how cancer patients in China communicate about their illness and how they gain social support when people do not want to talk about cancer."

She agreed with the importance of the topic and shared that she was hesitant to discuss her illness even in the United States, for fear that she would be considered "unlucky." She said that people did not know how to communicate with cancer patients and that Chinese people especially lack communication skills in relating to cancer patients. "I am not saying that Chinese folks have no sympathy. I just don't like the way people have that look like you are dying."

As we talked, Yijun opened up more about her thoughts throughout the past year: "When the doctor told me the diagnosis, I thought, 'Why me?' I take very good care of myself and eat healthily. I hardly consume meat in my diet, I exercise often, and no one in my family has had breast cancer." She said the size of her tumor had grown. She had been busy and stressed out at work in the past year and had skipped several important medical appointments. I asked her if she would mind if I consulted Meihua, who had scheduled surgery at a prominent university hospital at the end of January. Yijun hesitated but agreed.

I talked to Meihua and told her about Yijun's diagnosis and her unconventional treatment. Meihua told me about the doctors she visited and the surgeon she chose. She offered to take Yijun to the same doctors she visited.

I thanked Meihua and called Yijun. I strongly suggested she immediately visit a western oncologist to undergo conventional treatment. Yijun said she needed to think about it. A few weeks later, she told me that her decision to continue with alternative medicine had not changed.

Epiphany 3: Spiritual Healing, Friendship, and Family

Searching through my email, I found lots of email messages between Yijun and me from January 2011 to June 2012, most of which were forwarded messages and links about spiritual healing and church announcements of medical healing retreats. Yijun always said that she believed God had a plan for her sickness and that she believed in God's healing power. Whenever she felt her symptoms had improved, she praised God. She shared her diary with me and her daughter, Vivi; she asked me to translate some of the contents to her after Yijun passed away. In talking about faith and healing, I sometimes argued with Yijun, "Don't you think that God heals through the hands of doctors and nurses?" She would say, "I don't know how, but I do believe God heals." She did not seem to trust many people with her experience. For example, a family with whom she was good friends and attended the same church for many years, did not know about Yijun's illness until after her death.

In the summer of 2011, Meihua invited Yijun and me to a series of Christian Charismatic Healing Retreats. It was the first time the three of us met together after both of them came to know about each other's health conditions. At this particular healing retreat, I noticed Yijun looked weaker and thinner. The complexion on her face looked grayish. Because of their common experiences, I hoped she could discuss her cancer with Meihua freely. I also hoped that Meihua would be able to convince her to undergo conventional treatment. The two took a few private moments throughout the day. Meihua later told me that Yijun's situation had worsened and that the tumor in her breast had grown to the size of a fist. Yijun tired easily and left the retreat early.

In October 2011, Yijun finally told her sister and brother in China about her health condition. They urged her to go back to China as soon as possible. Her siblings knew some experts in renowned hospitals and offered to arrange an appointment with the hospital. It would be easier for family members to take care of her after the possible surgery. When I gave her a ride to the airport, she told me she agreed to go back to China because she admired traditional Chinese herbal medicine and believed there was an effective herbal treatment for cancer.

Epiphany 4: Advanced Stage of Cancer

I saw Yijun one month after she came back from China. The trip to China did not bring any good news. The Chinese oncologists evaluated her reports and said her tumor size was too large to operate on. One Sunday I gave her a ride to a newly established Chinese Christian church, where the pastor believes positive thinking and attitude will transform a person's life. We had met the pastor in a spiritual retreat. As soon as Yijun entered the car, I noticed a noxious odor. She told me the tumor had broken through her skin and that she had no idea what to do with it. "It was very, very bad."

Yijun's sister and brother in-law came to the United States to take care of her in December 2011. In the middle of January of 2012, Yijun called from the hospital to tell me that she went to the ER and was later admitted to the hospital because of massive bleeding from her cancer wounds.

I stepped into her hospital room, and I was almost forced back by an overwhelming stench. She was surrounded by her daughter, sister, and Maria, who I later learned was, other than me, the only friend who knew about her illness. The doctor had just finished discussing possible treatment options. Everyone in the room urged her to follow the doctor's order. Yijun thanked everyone for caring about her and apologized for being so stubborn. She said, "I should repent my sin to God for not listening to the physicians sooner. I'll listen to the doctors and start conventional treatment." She admitted that it was her fault to have missed the optimal treatment time. But hopefully, it was not too late. I read Yijun's medical report and felt embarrassed because I could not understand most of the medical terms on that report. I only recognized "metastasis." Cancer cells had spread to Yijun's liver, lungs, and lymph nodes. I suddenly understood why cancer patients in China were the last to know of their own illness. I wondered if I were that sick, would I really want to know the truth?

Epiphany 5: The Last Stage of Her Journey

Yijun started chemotherapy in February 2012. However, the results were not promising, and she concluded her last round of chemotherapy in April. Her sister and brother-in-law stayed with her for six months. They told me about their concerns for Yijun and the futility of the medical decisions she made previously. Vivi was a junior in college and was going to get a driver's license so she could drive her mother to the hospital.

In July 2011, Yijun's sister and brother-in-law went back to China. Shortly after, I called her and found out she was paralyzed and hospitalized. I drove to the hospital and found her lying on the bed. She was bald from the chemotherapy treatments by then but had a peaceful look on her face. She had collapsed in the bathroom the previous day and was rushed to the ER by ambulance. Cancer had spread to her spine and caused a fracture.

I found the courage to ask her about drafting a will, immediately adding, "Just to prepare for the worst, you know, to have peace of mind." Most Chinese people do not have a living will. It is a cultural barrier, as people think it is a curse to talk about a will when one is healthy and alive. To my relief, Yijun was not offended when I mentioned writing a will and actually thanked me for bringing it up. She then wrote down all the important account numbers and passwords for her daughter on a laptop.

Yijun updated the insurance beneficiary that day. The hospital procured for her a package of forms dealing with final wills, medical wills, and power of attorney, among other similar paperwork. Discussing living wills is always difficult for Chinese. The easy transition to the topic for Yijun surprised me. By then, her former pastor had come to know of her illness and had arranged several families to take turns to cook for her. I cooked several of her favorite dishes since she complained about the western food in the hospital.

A couple of days later, I received a call from Yijun. She asked me to look for a rehabilitation center for her. The hospital would discharge her after eight radiation treatments, and she would have to stay in a rehab center for recovery. The hospital provided a list of addresses of rehab facilities and hospices. The first rehabilitation center Vivi and I visited looked like a gym for recovering patients. We thought the second center was better since it had a hospice area as well. After speaking with the hospice manager, we decided it would be the better choice for Yijun.

When we told Yijun about the center, we had picked, and how it had both rehab and hospice facilities, Yijun objected. "Hospice is the place you go to wait to die! That's not the place I should go!" I dared not look at her. Did she still believe she had a chance to recover? She was not happy that the hospital wanted to discharge her that day since she had been hospitalized for ten days, the maximum amount of time she could stay according to her insurance policy. She felt that the hospital was in a hurry to discharge her. I negotiated with her case manager, and after consulting the insurance company, we were told that Yijun could stay another week until she finished all the prescribed radiation treatments.

By the time Yijun went to the hospice, it was August 2012. She had established a will and made me her will executive if something happened to her daughter. It was at that moment I felt both obliged and guilty. I did not realize until that moment that I was her only close friend till the end. The hospice did not provide any Chinese food, and she did not like to eat western food every day, so I prepared her favorite dishes each day. By then, only palliative treatment was given, and her health deteriorated at a visible pace. Yijun passed away on the morning of August 20, 2012, at age 56.

MAKING SENSE OF THE LOSS

For years I could not deal with the fact that Yijun had passed away. It was the first time I encountered death at such a close distance. Watching a friend die is difficult. I was in a constant emotional misery, anger, and regret. I am angry that she did not initially choose conventional treatment and remained silent and invisible during her battle. I regret that as one of her few close friends who knew of her condition, I was unable to convince her to make the "right choice." I am angry at the Chinese community, her church, her family members, and her friends for not offering good social support. I questioned if there was a "right choice" when it came to cancer. In recent years, as I encountered more and more people with cancer at various stages and of various types, I found myself inwardly pessimistic but obligated to be outwardly positive for their family members or friends. Since I have done cancer research, I am regarded by friends as "brave" and "competent in communicating with cancer patients." When someone's beloved one is diagnosed with cancer, my friends call me to be the informant. I have to remind everyone that I am not a medical professional, that I might know how to communicate and suggest how they might emotionally support a friend with cancer, but I do not know what caused cancer or how to treat cancer.

To answer the research questions proposed earlier: What contributed to the invisibility of those with breast cancer in the Chinese American group? What has silenced the community and prevents the patient from openly discussing breast cancer? What implications and recommendations can be gleaned from Yijun's lived experiences in fighting and losing this battle?

Cancer patients want emotional and social support from their loved ones. But usually, they fight a battle in isolation and silence. In the Chinese community, the gap between cancer patients and the healthy population/community is huge. This results in relational tensions. Cancer patients are usually frustrated and disappointed about the misunderstanding and so choose to keep thoughts and emotions to themselves. On the other side, the cancer patients' friends and family members are afraid that they might say the wrong things and upset the patients. So, they remain distant (Sun and Critchfield, 2012). It is important that both cancer patients and their loved ones receive proper training so that they can overcome communication barriers.

When making decisions about medical treatment, cancer patients need to be provided with all necessary treatment options and with guidance. Medical professionals and primary doctors of cancer patients should take initiatives to educate patients about treatment procedures. In Yijun's case, she chose alternative medicine for cancer treatment. A responsible oncologist would not have suggested that option. There is no scientific proof that alternative treatment can cure cancer. Furthermore, Li and his associates (2013) reviewed 2,964 clinical cases where Chinese traditional medicine was used to treat cancer and found that between 1984–2011, 72 percent of traditional medicine treatments were used in conjunction with conventional cancer treatments. Another study found out that 22 percent of Chinese American women used herbal remedies when diagnosed with breast cancer. The American Cancer Society warns that "it is a major problem." (Ernst and Cassileth, 1998). Other studies on the effectiveness of alternative medicine generated conflicting results (Ernst and Cassileth, 1998; Ernst, 1995).

Spiritual healing is regarded as part of alternative treatments, and scientists suggest that while it should not replace conventional medical treatment, it could have potential benefits in increasing patients' satisfaction (Shavers, Harlan and Stevens, 2003). The Chinese Christian community holds beliefs similar to the African American community regarding spirituality and healing (Madlock Gatison, 2016). Passages from the Bible, the pastor's relationship, and service offered to the patient, and congregational support is all important in keeping a cancer patient strong and feeling loved and supported.

As a single Chinese American mother, Yijun's choices of getting credible resources and generating a social support group were limited. This was partly due to her personality but also partly due to the neglect of her social circle. She also did not have an entrusted medical team to keep her informed and ensure all necessary treatments were followed. Finally, there was a lack of support from her employer in her battle against her illness.

Numerous studies have confirmed the important roles culture plays in effective health communication, "The cultural characteristics of any given group may be directly or indirectly associated with health-related priorities, decisions, behaviors, and/or with acceptance and adoption of health education and health communication programs and messages" (Kreuter and McClure, 2004, p. 440). Cultural appropriateness and cultural sensitivity have become the most important components of communication competencies in the healthcare profession (Kreuter and McClure, 2004; Thompson et al., 2008). To transmit health messages to different cultural groups, message creators need to consider different cultural characteristics. The Chinese culture is a collective, highly contextual, and gender-specific culture where harmonious relationships are valued. People tend to prefer to communicate indirectly. First generation Asian Americans encountered contradictions in all aspects of communication patterns to their own indigenous culture as they adapted to American life. The relationships and support systems, which are considered key aspects in cancer patients' survivorship, barely exist for Chinese American cancer patients. The relationships are challenged due to one person's illness. Within Chinese communities, the spiritual support that has been offered to African American patients and other cancer patients with a strong church community is only available to those who are Chinese Christians and faith seekers. Chinese speaking pastors are juniors in the service field and less experienced in providing spiritual healing strategies compared to their American counterparts. Adding to his desire to remain silent due to the fear to be rejected, the burden of dealing with a fatal disease often falls solely on the shoulders of a cancer patient. Madlock Gatison (2016) has found in her study that women with breast cancer are usually engaged in self-imposed silence. Minority women cancer patients and survivors are taking unnecessary burdens on this lonely journey.

The walls of invisibility in minority health care need to be broken down. It might take many years. Cancer patients' voices, stories, and life experiences need to be heard so that the public can come to understand what they have gone through and respond properly. The community as a whole needs to realize there is an urgency to raise awareness to the issue and to advocate, to educate, and to bring about change.

REFERENCES

Andreeva, V.A., Unger, J.B. and Pentz MA. (2007). "Breast cancer among immigrants: A systematic review and new research directions." *Journal of Immigrant Minor Health*, 9(4), 307–322.

Barrett, M., Chu, A., Chen, J., Dhingra, L. (2015). "Use of complementary and alternative medicine approaches for cancer pain management in Chinese-American immigrants." *Journal of Pain*, *16*(4), 112.

Bochner, A. P. (2012). "On first-person narrative scholarship: Autoethnography as acts of meaning." *Narrative Inquiry* , *22*(1), 155–164.

Byrd, R. C. (1988). "Positive therapeutic effects of intercessory prayer in coronary care unit population." *Southern Medical Journal*, *81*(7), 826–829.

Cheng, A. W., Chang, J., O'Brien, J. Budgazad, M. S. and Tsai, J. (2017). "Model minority stereotype: Influence on perceived mental health needs of Asian Americans." *Journal of Immigrant and minority Health*. *19*(3), 572–581.

DeSantis, C. E., Fedewa, S. A., Sauer, A. G., Kramer, J. L. Smith, R. A. and Jemal, A. (2015). "Breast cancer statistics, 2015: Convergence of incidence rates between black and white women." *CA: A Cancer Journal for Clinicians*, *66*(1), 31–42.

Dutta, M.J. (2007). "Communicating about culture and health: Theorizing culture-centered and cultural sensitivity approaches." *Communication Theory*, *17*(3), 304–328.

Ellis, C., Adams, T. E. and Bochner, A. P. (2010). "Autoethnografie." In Günter Mey and Katja Mruck (Eds.), *Handbuch Qualitative Forschung in der Psychologie* (pp.345–357). Wiesbaden: VS Verlag/Springer.

Ellis, C. and Bochner, A. P. (2000). "Autoethnography, personal narrative, reflexivity." In K. Denzin & Y. S. Lincoln (Eds.), *Handbook of qualitative research* (2nd ed., pp.733–768). Thousand Oaks, CA: Sage.

Ellis, C. and Bochner, A.P. (2006). "Analyzing analytic autoethnography: An autopsy." *Journal of Contemporary Ethnography*, *35*(4), 429–449.

Ernst, E. (1995). "Complementary cancer treatments: Hope or hazard?" *Clinical Oncology*, *7*(4), 259–263.

Ernst E. and Cassileth, B.R. (1998). "The prevalence of complementary/alternative medicine in cancer: A systematic review. *Cancer*, *83*(4), 777–782.

Ferrante, J.M., Chen, P.H. and Kim, S. (2008). "The effect of patient navigation on time to diagnosis, anxiety, and satisfaction in urban minority women with abnormal mammograms: A randomized controlled trial." *Journal of Urban Health*, *85*(1), 729–734.

Ferrante, J.M., Wu, J. and Dicicco-Bloom, B. (2011). "Strategies used and challenges faced by a breast cancer patient navigator in an urban underserved community." *Journal of the National Medical Association, 103*(8), 729–734.

Frisby, C. M. (2002). "Health communication strategies that address barriers preventing black women from screening for breast cancer." *Journal of Black Studies*, *32*(5), 489–505.

Giaconomi, G., Venturini, E., Hoarau, H., Guyon, F. and Conri, V. (2014). "How women with gynaecological cancer deal with treatment: Issues of visibility and invisibility." *Gynécologie Obstétrique & Fertilité* , *42*(11), 795–799.

Hofmann, A. R. (2004). "Visibility and invisibility of organs in women and their influence on the perception of illness." *Junctures*, *3*, 43–57.

Kien, G. (2013). "The nature of epiphany." *International Review of Qualitative Research, 6*(4), 578–584.

Kreuter, M. W. and McClure, S. M. (2004). "The role of culture in health communication." *Public Health, 25, 439–455.*

Lee, M. M, Lin S.S., Wrensch, M. R., Adler S. R. and Eisenberg, D. (2000). "Alternative therapies used by women with breast cancer in four ethnic populations." *Journal of the National Cancer Institute, 92*(1), 42–47.

Lent, R. W. (2007). "Restoring emotional well-being: A theoretical model." In M. Feuerstein. (Ed.). *Handbook of cancer survivorship,* 231–248. New York: Springer.

Li, X., Yang, G., Li, X., Zhang, Y., Yang, J., Chang, J., Sun, X., Zhou, X., Guo,Y., Xu, Y., Liu, J. and Bensoussan, A. (2013). "Traditional Chinese medicine in cancer care: A review of controlled clinical studies published in Chinese." *PLoS One, 8(4), e60338.*

Liao, K., Yeung, N., Wong, C., Warmoth, K. and Lu, Q. (2017). "Fear of cancer recurrence and physical well-being among Chinese cancer survivors: The role of conscientiousness, positive reappraisal and hopelessness." *Supportive Care in Cancer. 25* (4), 1141–1149.

Long, L. (2008). "Narrative autoethnography and the promotion of spiritual well-being in teacher research and practice." *Pastoral Care in Education*, *26* (3), 187–196.

Luhar, M. (2015). Plum blossoms aims to empower Asian American women with breast cancer." *NBCNews,* October 26, 2015.

Madlock Gatison, A.D. (2016). *Health communication and breast cancer among Black women: culture, identity, spirituality and strength.* Landover, MD: Lexington Books.

Nicolaisen A., Hansen, D. G., Hagedoorn, M., Flyger, H. E., Rottmann, N., Nielsen, P. Soe, K., Pedersen, A. E. and Johansen, C. (2014). "Attachment-oriented psychological intervention for couples facing breast cancer: Protocol of a randomised controlled trial." *BCM Psychology*, *1*(2), 10–19.

Orbe, M. P. (1998). *Constructing co-cultural theory: An explication of culture, power and communication.* Thousand Oaks, CA: Sage.

Shavers, V.L., Harlan, L.C. and Stevens, J.L. (2003). "Racial/ethnic variation in clinical presentation, treatment, and survival among breast cancer patients under age 35." *Cancer, 97*(1):134–147.

Sun, W. (2007). *Minority Invisibility: An Asian American experience.* The University of Press of America.

Sun, W. and Crtichfield, A.J. (2012). "Inoculating Invisibility and communicating cancer among survivors, health providers and caregivers: The Friendly Circle of Cancer Patients Chinese blog." In P. H. Cheong, J. Martin and L. Macfadyen (Eds.). *New Media and Intercultural Communication.* Peter Lang.

Sun, W. and Starosta, W. J. (2006). "Perceptions of minority invisibility among Asian American professionals." *Howard Journal of Communications*, *17*(2). 119–142.

Thompson, S., Cavazos-Rehg, P.A., K., Jupkal, K., Cayton, N., Gratzke, J., Tate, K.Y., Deshpande, A. and Kreuter, M.W. (2008). "Evidential preferences: cultural appropriateness strategies in health communications." *Health Education Research*, *23*(3), 549–559.

Waldrop, D.P., O'Connor, T.L., Trabold, N. (2011). "Waiting for the other shoe to drop: Distress and coping during and after treatment for breast cancer." *Journal of Psychosocial Oncology, 29*, 450–473.

Williams, F. and Jeanetta, S. (2016). "Lived experiences of breast cancer survivors after diagnosis, treatment and beyond: Qualitative study." *Health Expect*, *19*(3): 631–642.

Index

About the Editors and Contributors

Nicole Defenbaugh is an associate professor at Morsani College of Medicine—USF and the Director of Education for the Department of Family Medicine at Lehigh Valley Health Network. She is a state and national speaker on chronic illness identity and was the national spokesperson for Celebrating UC (ulcerative colitis) in 2010. She has presented and performed at various health organizations including Baylor University, Penn State College of Medicine—Hershey, Penn State Medical and Geisinger (Danville, PA). Nicole has won the Outstanding Specialist Educator Award (2016), Norman K. Denzin Qualitative Research Award (2011), and Ellis-Bochner Autoethnography and Personal Narrative Research Award (2009). She has a single-authored book titled, *Dirty Tale: A Narrative Journey of the IBD Body* (2011, Hampton) and articles in the *Journal of Graduate Medical Education, Journal of Health Communication, Qualitative Inquiry, International Review of Qualitative Research, Nursing Education in Practice* and an upcoming co-authored autoethnographic piece in the *Annals of Family Medicine*.

Elizabeth Desnoyers-Colas is an associate professor of communication at Armstrong State University, Savannah Georgia. Academe is Elizabeth Desnoyers-Colas's second career. She spent fifteen years of military service as an Air Force Public Affairs Relations Officer and was awarded the Defense Meritorious Service Medal upon her retirement from active duty in 1995. Her military duties time included serving as a speechwriter for senior DOD military and civilian officials on EEO/EEO related issues, operating as the director of the Joint Task Force Information Bureau, Haitian Refugee Humanitarian Rescue Effort, and Guantanamo Bay, Cuba. She also served in Operation Desert Storm and was deployed to Central Air Forces, Forward, Dhahran, Saudi Arabia, as the Director of Public Affairs/Protocol, Operation Desert

Storm. Currently, her research interests focus on how African Americans use story-telling and narrative as an integral cultural oral communication tool to gather and preserve oral histories of their military service during combat and peacetime.

Laura L. Ellingson is a professor of communication and women's and gender studies at Santa Clara University. Her passion for methodological and epistemological innovation infuses all of her research and creative work. She seeks to enlarge possibilities for spanning theoretical, paradigmatic, and representational boundaries through her development of a crystallization framework for qualitative research (*Engaging Crystallization in Qualitative Research*, 2009, Sage) and her articulation of embodied research strategies (*Embodiment in Qualitative Research,* 2017, Routledge). Narrative, feminist, and pragmatic perspectives guide her ethnographic research in communication in health care delivery and in extended/chosen families. In addition to numerous articles and chapters, she is the author of *Communicating in the Clinic: Negotiating Frontstage and Backstage Teamwork* (2005, Hampton) and co-author with Dr. Patty Sotirin of *Aunting: Cultural Practices that Sustain Family and Community Life* (2010, Baylor University Press) and *Where the Aunts Are: Family, Feminism, and Kinship in Popular Culture* (2013, Baylor University Press).

Eletra S. Gilchrist-Petty is an associate professor of communication arts at The University of Alabama Huntsville. Her programs of research focus on instructional communication, interpersonal communication, and African American communication from both the quantitative and qualitative perspectives. Gilchrist-Petty is the author of *Deviant Communication in Teacher-Student Interactions: Emerging Research and Opportunities* (in press, IGI Global). She is also the editor of *Experiences of Single African-American Women Professors: With this PhD, I Thee Wed* (2011, Lexington Books), and she is the co-editor of *Contexts of the Dark Side of Communication* (2016, Peter Lang). She has also published in many leading scholarly outlets, including *Review of Communication, Journal of Intercultural Communication Research, Communication Reports, Journal of the National Academic Advising Association (NACADA), NIDA Journal of Language and Communication, Communication Teacher*, *Southern Communication Journal,* and *The Northwest Journal of Communication.*

Cerise L. Glenn is an associate professor in the department of communication studies at the University of North Carolina at Greensboro (UNCG). She is the program director of the African American and African Diaspora Studies Program at UNCG. Additionally, she is the faculty fellow of the University Faculty Mentoring Program. Her research interests center on social constructions of difference (diversity), particularly identity negotiation and representations of underrepresented groups in educational, workplace, intercultural/international, and mass-mediated contexts. She has published in edited books and journals, including the *Journal of Black Studies*, the *Howard Journal of Communications*, *Sexuality & Culture*, and *Continuum: Journal of Media & Cultural Studies*. She is currently editing a special issue of *Women and Language* titled "Michelle Obama: Feminism and the First Lady of the United States."

Annette Madlock Gatison is an associate professor of communication and women's studies at Southern Connecticut State University. Her primary research interests explore social activism, health, and media as it relates to black women's health both globally and domestically. Her work explores issues of identity, family and work life balance, policy, and socioeconomic factors are explored through content, discourse, and thematic analysis as well as focus groups, interviews, and survey methods. To ground and inform her research an applied approach Dr. Madlock Gatison serves on Breast Cancer Consortium Advisory Board; an international partnership committed to the scientific and public discourse about breast cancer that promotes collaborative initiatives among researchers, advocates, health professionals, educators, and others who focus on the systemic factors that impact breast cancer as an individual experience, a social problem, and a health epidemic. She is also a graduate of the National Breast Cancer Coalition's Project L.E.A.D., which is an intensive science institute taught by renowned research faculty covering the basics.

Frances "Selena" Morant is a psychiatric nurse with an assertive community treatment (ACT) program; a team-based treatment model that provides multidisciplinary, flexible treatment and support to people with mental illness 24/7 in Tampa, FL. She currently holds a master's degree in counseling and is presently working toward a second master's degree in public health. She plans to work in underserved populations emphasizing the importance of physical, emotional, and mental health on the development of the total healthy self. She began experiencing lupus symptoms in college in the early nineties, but the symptoms were not identified as lupus during that time. Selena was diagnosed with lupus in December 2005; shortly after finishing nursing school and accepting a nursing position at a Veterans' Hospital. Her work was most recently published in *American Family Physician.*

Emily Pfender is a graduate student in the department of communication at Villanova University. She is also a graduate assistant at the Office of Diversity. During her graduate studies, she intends to do more autoethnographic work that explores Borderline Personality Disorder, which she was diagnosed with in 2015. Other research interests include disability culture, mental illness, well-being, storytelling, and interpersonal communication. As a communication arts and sciences undergraduate student at Penn State University, Berks, Emily presented research at the Eastern Communication Association Conference that works to encourage those suffering from mental health disorders to disclose their illnesses to professors, family members, and friends in an effort to be more successful throughout their undergraduate studies, all of which stems from personal experience.

Launick Saint-Fort is a post-baccalaureate fellow currently investigating the potential heterogeneity in smoking behavior among US blacks in relation to immigration status and country of birth. Through this research, she hopes to contribute to current efforts in reducing health disparities in black populations by providing data that can be used to develop intervention and prevention methods representative of the diversity within the black community. Prior to her fellowship, Saint-Fort attended Penn State Berks as a Schreyer Scholar and received a bachelor in biochemistry and molecular biology. Saint-Fort's research inquiries have been heavily influenced by her childhood in Haiti, her experiences as a first generation immigrant, and a keen interest in the many factors presently affecting black communities around the world. Following her unprecedented diagnosis with postural orthostatic tachycardia syndrome, Saint-Fort transitioned from a traditional wet lab to social and behavioral epidemiology to explore the effects of behavior on health, particularly, within marginalized populations.

Wei Sun is a graduate faculty at department of communication, culture and media studies, Howard University. Her research interests include intercultural communication, media studies, health communication, and minority invisibility. She teaches intercultural communication, qualitative research methods, social media, communication and culture, diversity and leadership, etc. Her publications have appeared in *The Howard Journal of Communications*, *Intercultural Communication Studies*, and *World Communication.* Her scholarly works have been included in several books. Her book *Minority Invisibility: an Asian American Experience* was published in 2007.

Hannah Thyberg is a registered nurse working in the Pittsburgh area. She is a graduate of the Templeton Honors College at Eastern University where she received a bachelor of arts in communication studies. After completing her undergraduate degree, Hannah went back to school and obtained a bachelor of science in nursing through the University of Pittsburgh's School of Nursing accelerated second-degree program. She has been working in the field of pediatric and neonatal nursing since February 2015, in both hospital and homecare settings. Hannah's passion for medical advocacy began in early high school and was further fueled by her own experience with chronic illness. Diagnosed with Fibromyalgia in 2008, Hannah has spent the last decade working to hone her setbacks into strengths to provide holistic and compassionate care to her patients and families. This will be Hannah's first book publication, but her writing was previously featured in *Catapult Magazine.*

Kesha Morant Williams is an associate professor of communication arts and sciences at Penn State University, Berks. Her research interest focuses on interpersonal relationships, health communication, and popular media examined through a cultural lens. Her research has been published in peer review journals including *Journal of Health Communication, Journal of Medical Humanities, Journal of Black Studies, Howard Journal of Communications, Journal of Media and Religion, Journal of Communication & Religion, Sexuality and Culture, Journal of Contemporary Rhetoric,* and the books *Inter/ Cultural Communication: Representation and construction of culture in everyday interaction*, and *Race, Gender & Identity*. She is a featured scholar in the documentary *Beautiful Me*. Dr. Williams teaches courses including research methods, popular culture, interpersonal, family, and health communication.

Lightning Source UK Ltd.
Milton Keynes UK
UKHW02n1514220118
316629UK00003B/37/P

9 781498 551007